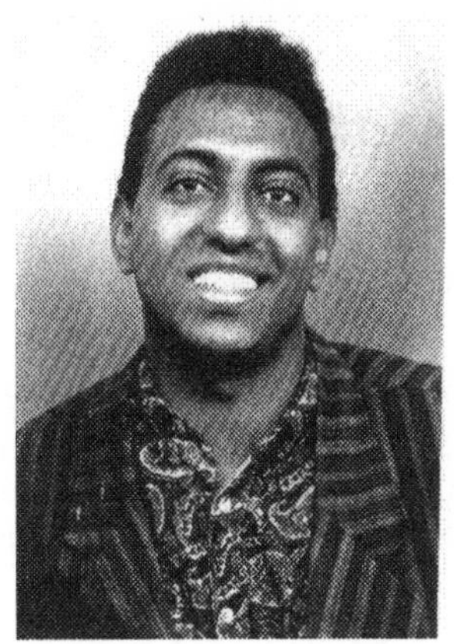

Teferra Haile-Giorgis

Published by
Chipmunkapublishing
PO Box 6872
Brentwood
Essex CM13 1ZT
United Kingdom

First published 2005

A record of this book is in the British Library.

This is a book of LOVE the features and design are kept form those submitted to the publisher out of respect.

http://www.chipmunkapublishing.com

The development of this book was made possible by a grant from The Arts Council, London.

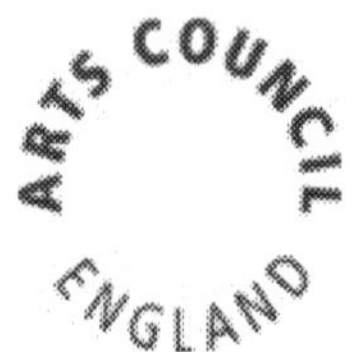

Table of Content

Abi's Biography 7th year memorial

6. **First Report Card**

7. **Abi's work of art (3 photos)**

8. **Abi with his parents (older child)**

9. **Abi at the palace (a picture with the Emperor at Christmas)**

10. **Abi with his father:**

    a. **Early childhood**

    b. **3 weeks before both died**

11. **Photos whilst parents were in prison**

12. **Report Cards**

    a) SANDFORD English Community School

    b) Seventh Day Adventist, Akaki School: 6th grade, 7th grade, 8th grade

    c) National Exams: Results for grade 6 and 8

13. **Abi with father and uncle David at Dean Close School (4 photos)**

14. The first letter to mother from school in the U.K and second and third letters 1984 placed in between to mother from Dean Close School

15. The first report from Dean Close School (2 pages)

16. Sport achievement (Marathon award for Dean Close School and Cheltenham) (3 photos)

17. Abi with families he lived with in the U.K at Christmas.

18. 2 photos with family

    a) At home in Addis Ababa

    b) At home in Manchester at Christmas, when mother was studying in Manchester.

19. Letters from Dean Close at different times placed in different places- To father and mother (1987, 1989)

20. Report cards for Spring Term before A level, and school report last summer term 1989.

21. **Holidays during mother's years in the U.K 1986-89 with children visit to Paris, Switzerland/ Lausanne, Geneva, Frankfurt/Cologn, Helsinki, Vienna etc.**
22. **Lancashire University (earlier Lancashire Polytechnic) where Abi started quantity Surveying (HND in Building Studies). Discontinued after 2 years due to illness.**
23. **Letter whilst at Lancashire Polytechnic (Lancashire University)**
24. **Abi with his brother and mother in Manchester 1988**
25. **Abi with his brother at different places (4 pictures)**
26. **Abi with his sisters (3 pictures)**
27. **Abi with his father and brother (2 pictures)**
28. **Abi alone (3 pictures)**
29. **The bed sit from where he lived in solitude**

30. **Abi Appealing to God also different concepts of God scribbled on one page during mental illness**
31. **Abi's diagnosis of illness**
32. **The 15 story office building (the Guild Hall) from which Abi took his life.**
33. **The Lancashire Evening Post announcement of Abi's death (2 pages)**
34. **Death certificate**
35. **Photos of tomb**
36. **Letters of condolence**
37. **The last photo together with his dad alive (Dad and son) 3 weeks before they both died**

Preface

"For Whom the Bell Tolls"

We never know what it feels like to be with the Good Lord, where we have no more earthly cares to worry about. I hope, somehow, that those who have left us to be with Him can see or know that their past concerns are addressed and their wishes have been fulfilled.

What was worrying our beloved Abi, at the last session in the hospital consulting room, at the Royal Preston Hospital, Avondale Unit, where we were sitting for group discussion? I clearly remember what the Psychiatrist said: "I am afraid your son's case does not fit into a 'British black' or a 'British white mental illness category' ".I can just remember my son abruptly getting up, being very angry and rushing to the door, then opening it and turning towards me before walking out. I can still hear him saying "You are wasting your time, Emmama, these people are dummies. I have repeatedly told you that they do not understand my case. I think that, if I ever get healed, I will help other victims like myself. It will only be someone like me, who has been through such illness that can help those in similar circumstances". He was not only concerned for himself, but for all others in similar circumstances. He obviously had a burning desire to be in a position to help those victims of political conflict, political imprisonment, displacement and other human suffering such as escapees, like himself, from enforced conscription. In today's world we are told that some 20 or more wars officially or unofficially go on in different parts of the world. Therefore, there must surely be more and more Abis whose pain, agony and depression and other related mental health problems are not understood or dismissed by the ordinary mental health services and psychiatrists.

Abi, very unfortunately, has suddenly chosen to leave us, by taking his own life. We will always feel hurt and upset, and will cherish his memory whenever we think how much pain, agony and suffering have caused this action. But we can still save many of them who are in his 'category'. We, as a family, have felt committed to his cause. Within our limitation we can, at least, address his concern by setting up a Trust to help carry out research which will result in attention being given and focusing on victims of wars, political conflicts, political imprisonment, enforced conscriptions and displacement as well as any direct or indirect problems related to these situations.

Abi, who has enabled this concern to be addressed, is challenging us today. May God help us to voice his grievances, be advocates for his cause, and promote ideas, to challenge the mental health institutions and psychiatrists, at all levels, to listen to voices of such victims and not be dismissive as Abi's Psychiatrists were. In his death he challenges us all today, as we set up this Trust for all the neglected and misunderstood thousands whose human rights agendas had never been addressed in any meaningful way. Abi challenges us even in his death. May God almighty let him know that even though he is gone those who have suffered like him will get relief in the future- however few or however many. May God make Abi's dream a reality. Then ***for him the bells will toll*** to congratulate him for including us in his endeavor.

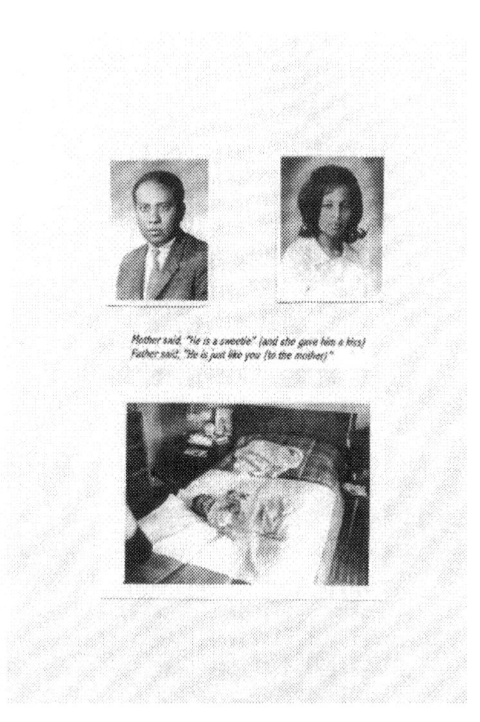

Mother said, "He is a sweetie" (and she gave him a kiss)
Father said, "He is just like you (to the mother)"

"….Mary said unto him, I know that he shall rise again in the resurrection at the last day. Jesus said unto her, I am the resurrection and the life: he that believe in me though he die yet shall he live". John 11:25

Seventh Year Remembrance for

Teferra Hailegiorgis
July 28th 1970 – September 20th 1996

Name: Teferra Hailegiorgis

Father: Dr. Workneh Hailegiorgis

Mother: Dr. Jember Teferra

Brother: Workneh Hailegiorgis

Sisters: - Memmenasha Hailegiorgis

- Lelo Hailegiorgis

Teferra, who was nicknamed "Abi" by his older brother, was born on July 28th 1970 or Hamley 21st 1962, according to the Ethiopian calendar. He was born at 9:45 pm in the Princess Tsehay hospital with Dr. Hamlin attending. Abi had been delivered on the day that he had been expected. He weighed 7lbs 90z and there had been no delivery complications. On the 40th day, according to the Ethiopian

Orthodox Judo- Christian tradition, he was baptized by Aba Girma Tseyon and Deacon Zenaw at Meskahezunan Medhanealem Church.

NAME.

DATE. 21/11/62

TIME.

DELIVERY. Normal

SEX. Male.

WEIGHT.

UNIT.

Hospital Birth Detail

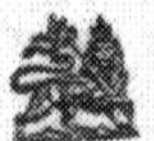

ቁጥር ....
No.

PRINCESS TSEHAI MEMORIAL HOSPITAL & SCHOOL

P. O. Box 1377

Telephone 47112-13

አዲስ ፡ አበባ ።
ADDIS ABABA

ADDIS ABABA ....19....

ለወላጆች የሚሰጥ የምስክር ወረቀት ።

BIRTH CERTIFICATE

This is to certify that woizero (Mrs) ....

gave birth to a living .....Male..... child ....

at this hospital on .....29. 7. 1970.....

Signed

Stamp.

ቀን .....6 · 9 · 1970

Date of Signature

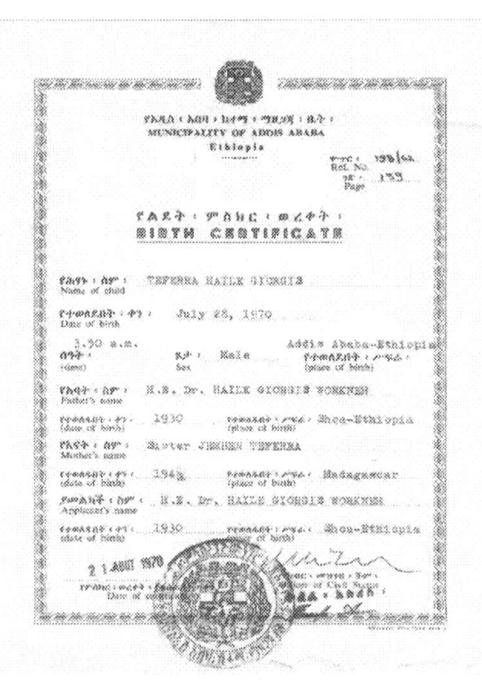

MUNICIPALITY OF ADDIS ABABA
Ethiopia

Ref. No. 198/64
Page 153

የልደት ፡ ምስክር ፡ ወረቀት ፡
BIRTH CERTIFICATE

Name of child: TEFERRA HAILE GIORGIS

Date of birth: July 28, 1970

(time) 3.50 a.m. Sex: Male (place of birth) Addis Ababa-Ethiopia

Father's name: H.E. Dr. HAILE GIORGIS WORKNEH

(date of birth) 1930 (place of birth) Shoa-Ethiopia

Mother's name: Sister JEMBER TEFERRA

(date of birth) 1945 (place of birth) Madagascar

Applicant's name: H.E. Dr. HAILE GIORGIS WORKNEH

(date of birth) 1930 (place of birth) Shoa-Ethiopia

21 AUG 1970

Date of [illegible]

[illegible] of Civil Status

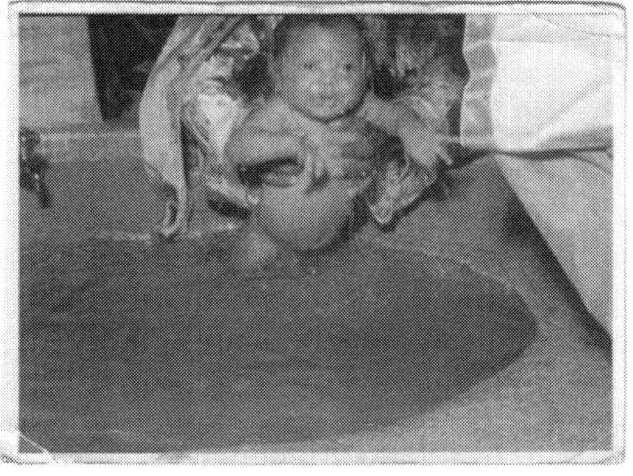

Abi at Christening

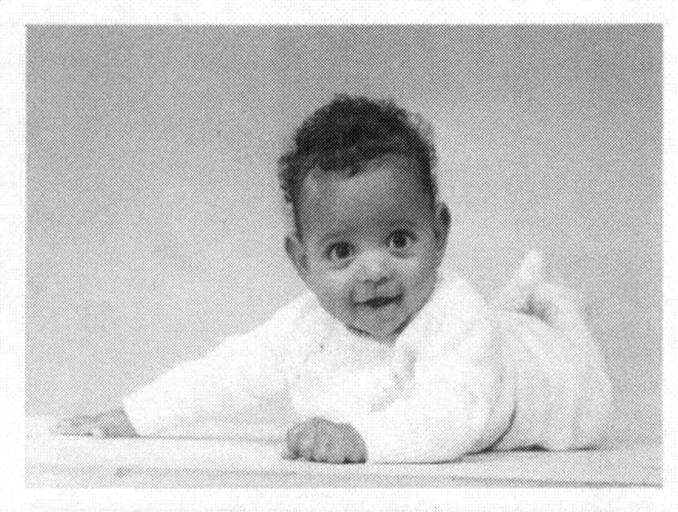

Teferra Hailegiorgis (later nicknamed Abi by his brother)

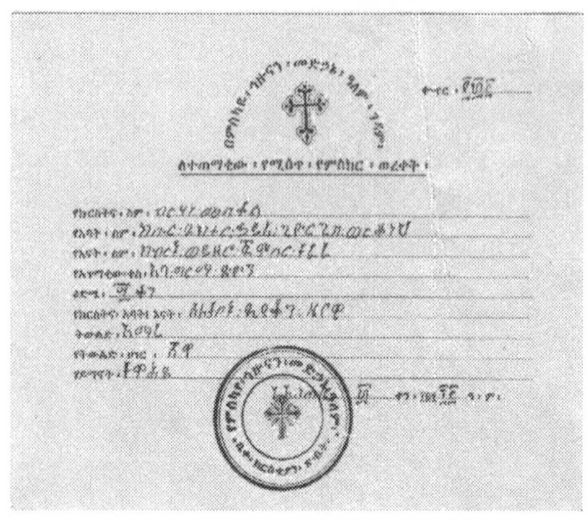

Certificate of Baptism

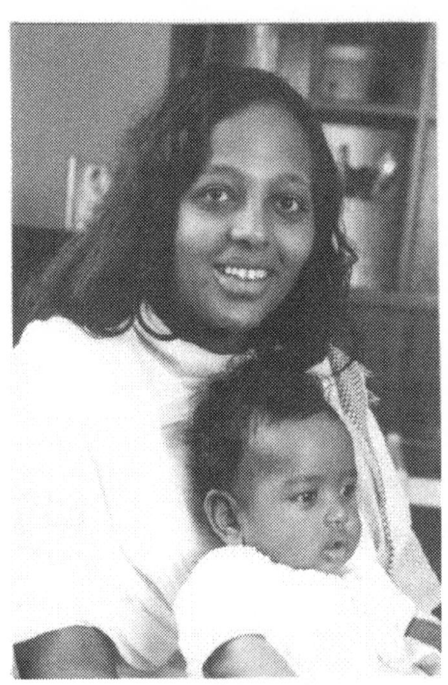

Abi with mother

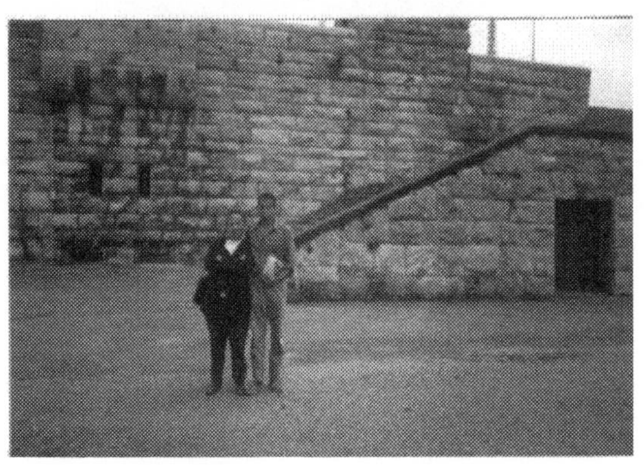

Abi with mother

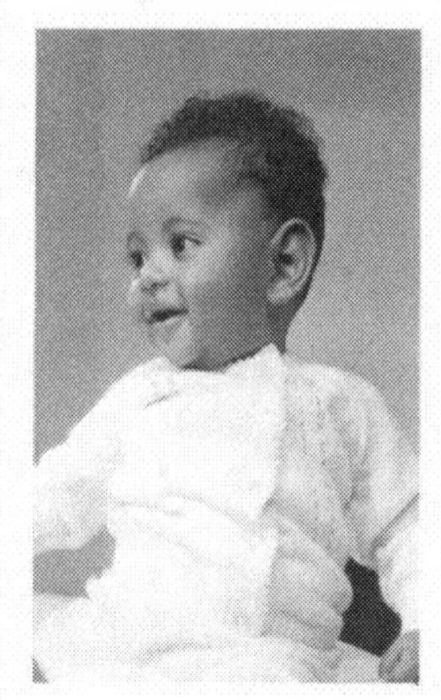

Childhood Picture

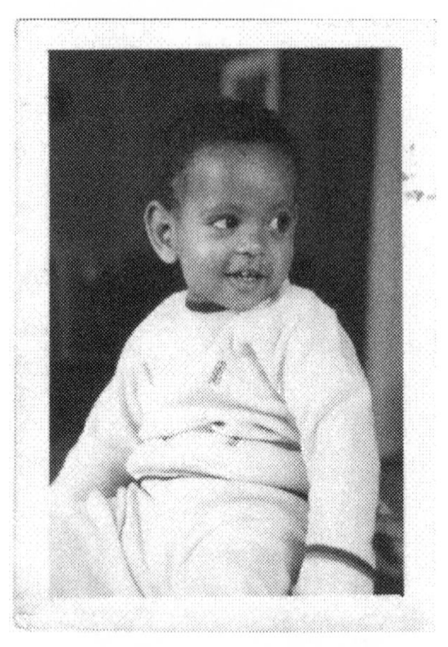

Childhood Picture

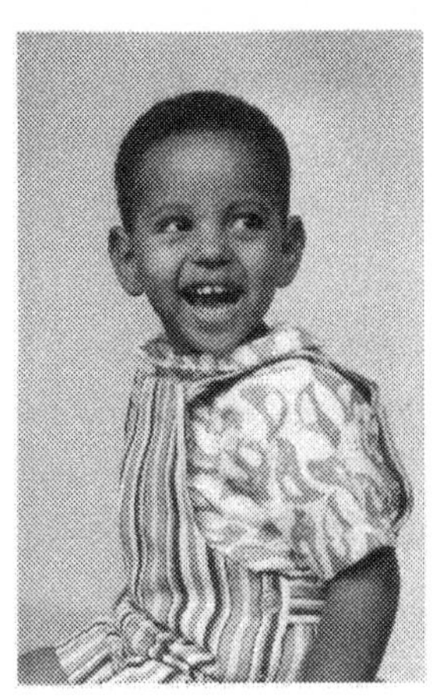

Childhood Picture

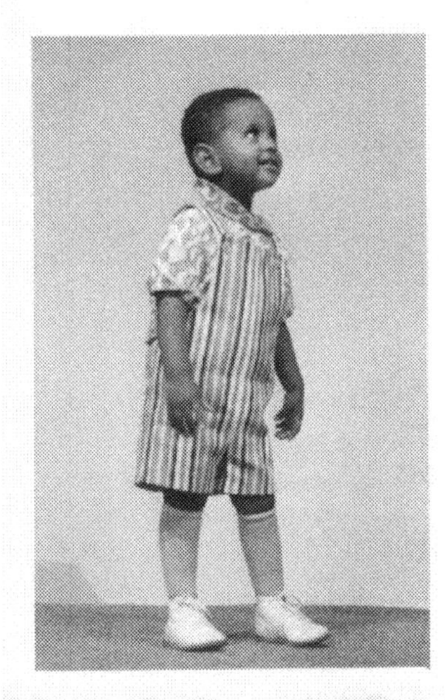

Childhood Picture

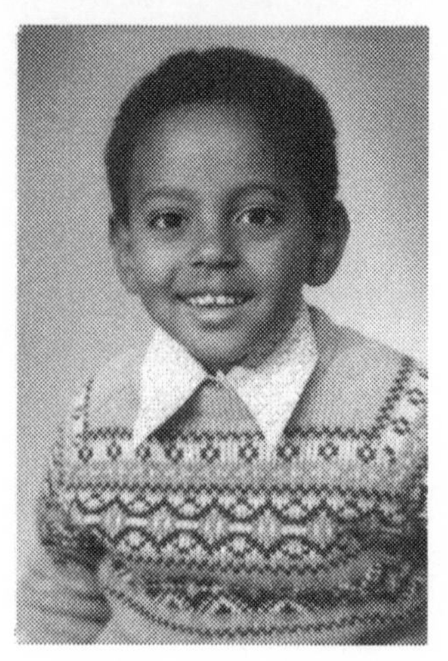

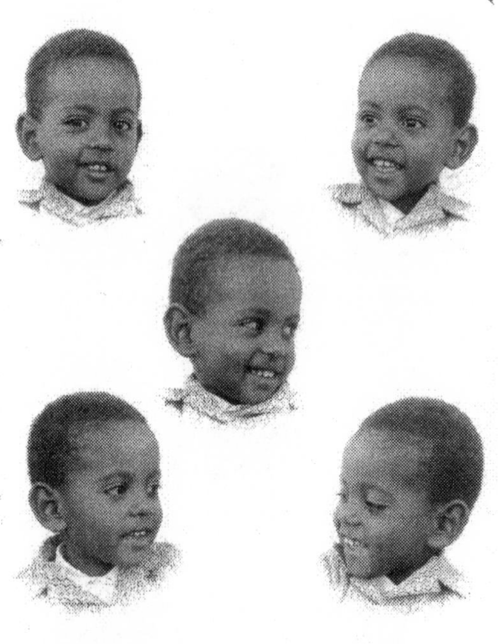

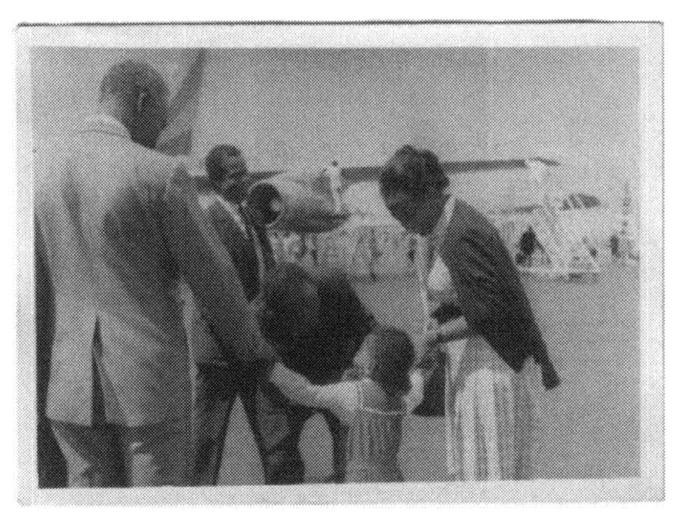

Abi with his mother and father

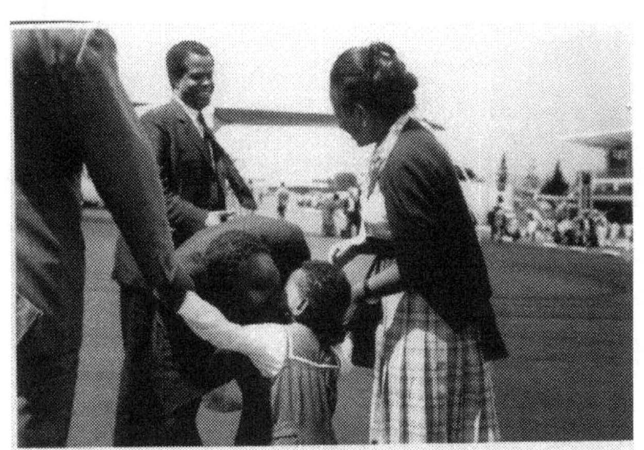

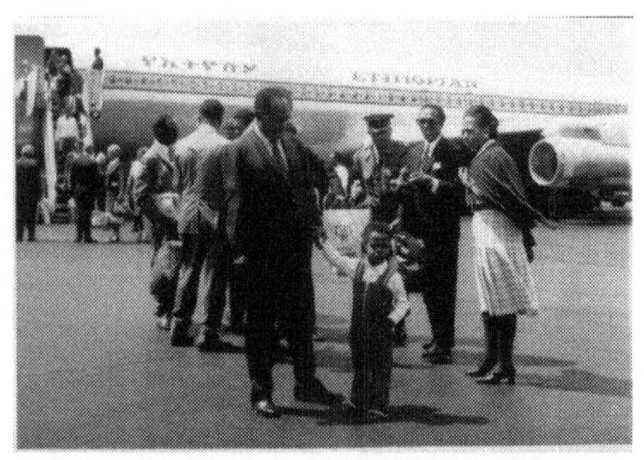

Abi with his mother and father

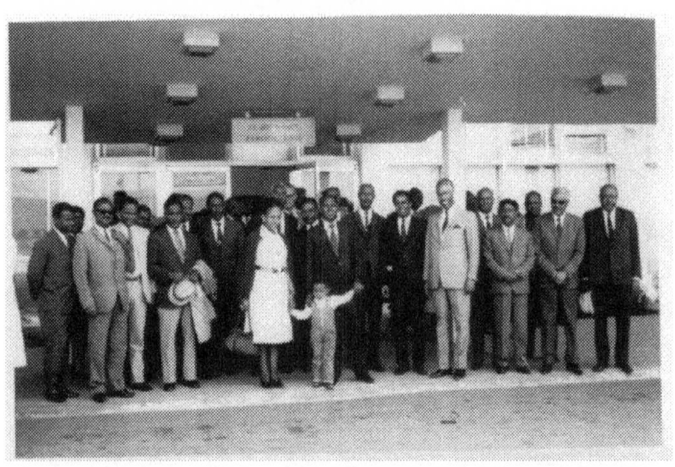

Abi with his mother and father

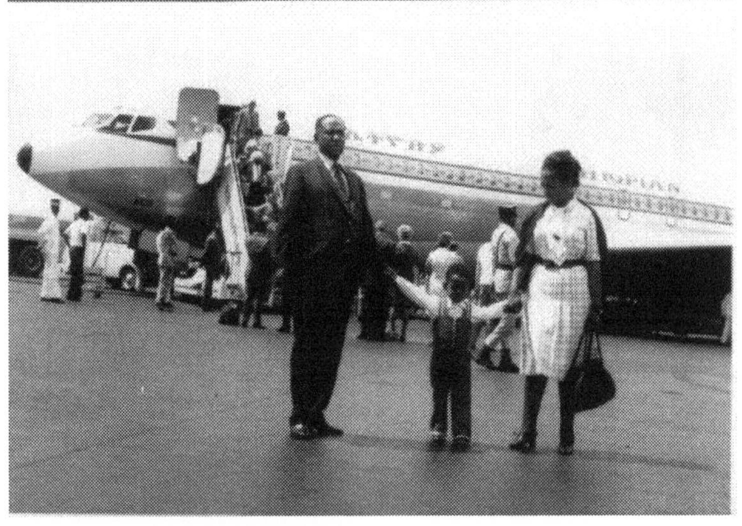

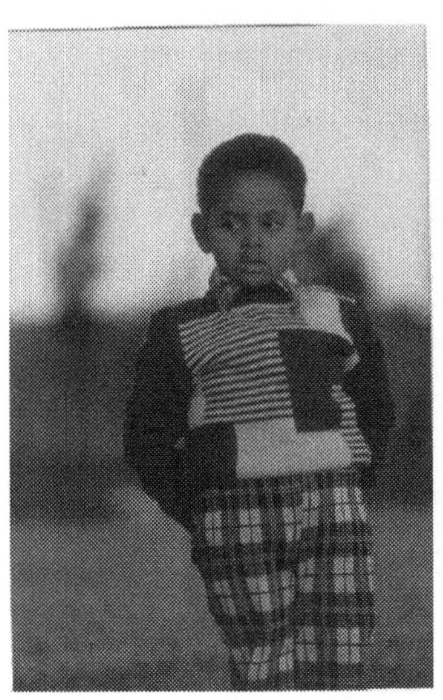

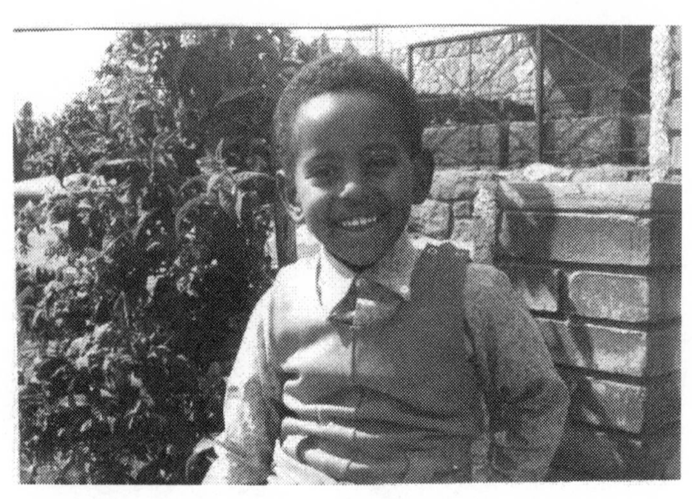

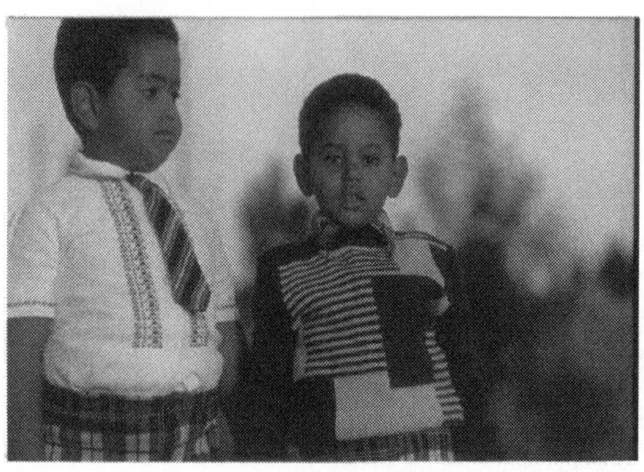

Abi with his brother

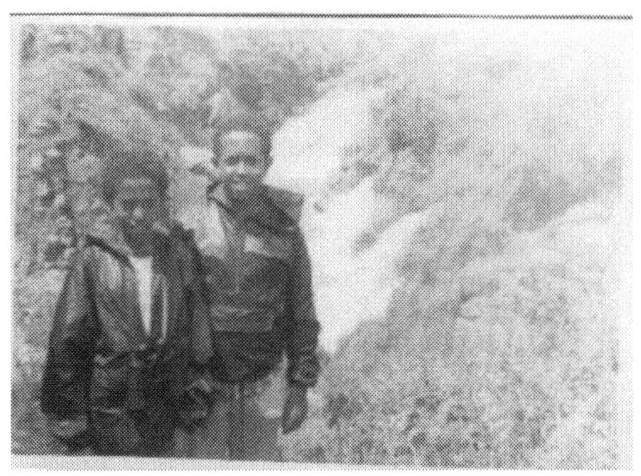

Abi with his brother

Abi had a happy childhood growing up with his brother, Workneh, who he was close to. When Workneh started to attend "Jack and Jill" Kindergarten, Abi had felt lonely and would spend his days by the river at the bottom of our garden playing with our three dogs Leon, Ambes and Menligodu. At a young age, he learnt to be good at enjoying his own company. As a child he was quick, observant and was able to assert himself when voicing things he felt very strongly about. By the time he joined his brother at the kindergarten he had been able to express his opinions about teachers and classmates in an open way. He was known to be cheeky at school and he expected all of us to accept his moments of naughtiness at home without too much fuss! If I smacked him lightly he would cry a little, roll his big lovely eyes and would ask in childish manner, “my tears are rolling down my face, what will that benefit you?” His teachers at Jack and Jill generally liked him. However, his father and I used to remember an incident at Jack and Jill where Abi had upset a teacher as a result of having spent the whole day making his classmates laugh and had made it impossible for the teacher to control the classroom.

Half way through Abi’s second year, at “Jack and Jill“, a Marxist revolution broke out in Ethiopia. Hailegiorgis was the Mayor of Addis Abeba. At that particular time existing officials were targets for imprisonment. Both boys could not attend school, for safety reasons, and ended up finishing their school that year with a private tutor .

Abi in a play at Christmas whilst in grade 1

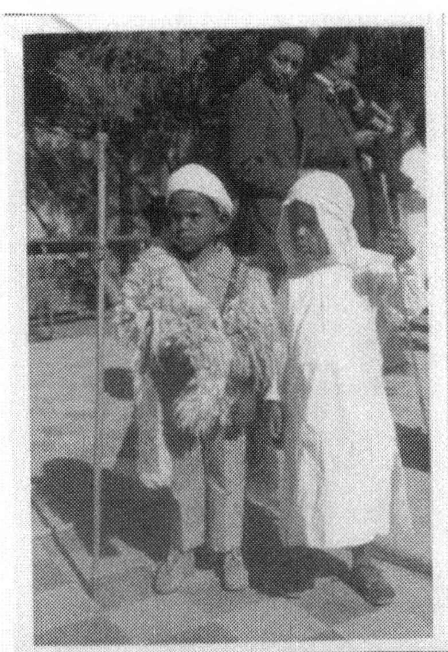

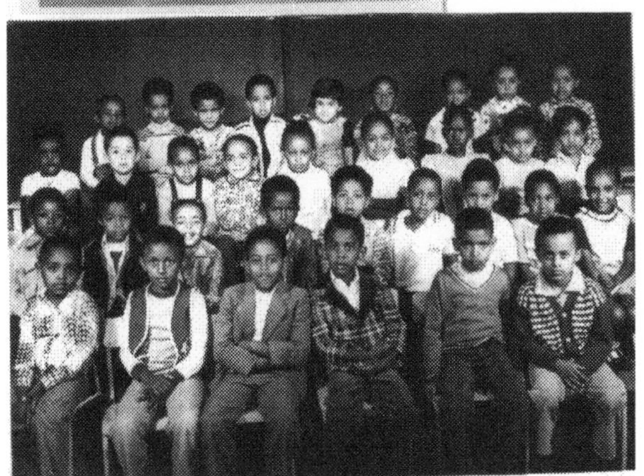

School photos

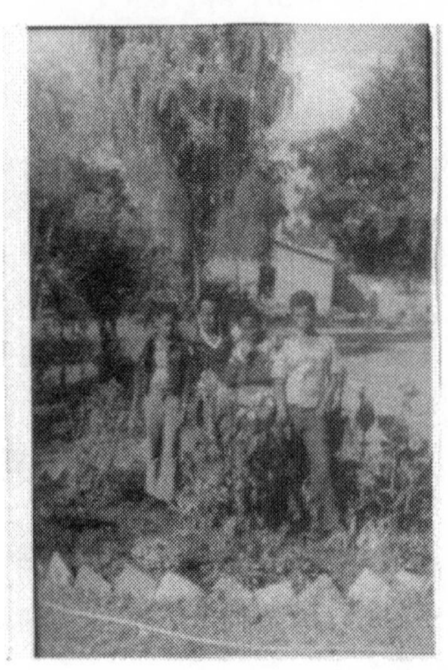

School photos

Date Feb 6th 1974

BEHAVIOUR PATTERN

Trefenna has settled down much better this term and seems to be very happy.

He has a number of friends and loves to play in a group. He shows no dependence on me or on any other child and always decides himself precisely what he wishes to do.

During formal parts of the morning Trefenna is cooperative and enjoys activities involving the whole class.

Date Feb 6th 1974

WORK HABITS

Trefenna is sometimes distracted by the attractions of play but can concentrate when he wishes.

He speaks very little English but obviously understands it well. When he does use English it is to sing to himself which he does most of the time.

He can count and knows differences in colour and shape.

He plays boisterously in the playground and shows good physical coordination.

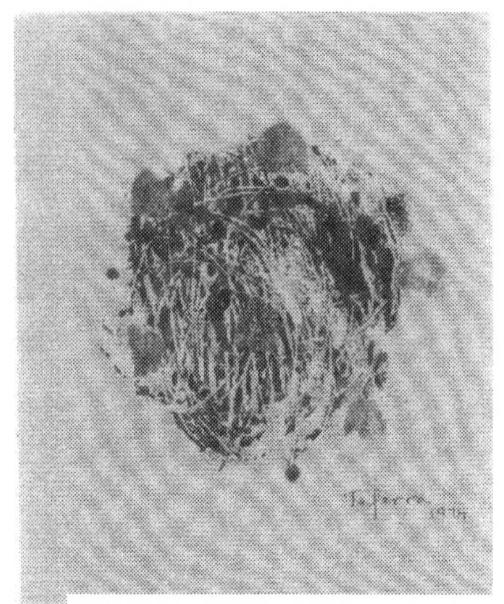

Some of Abi's art work

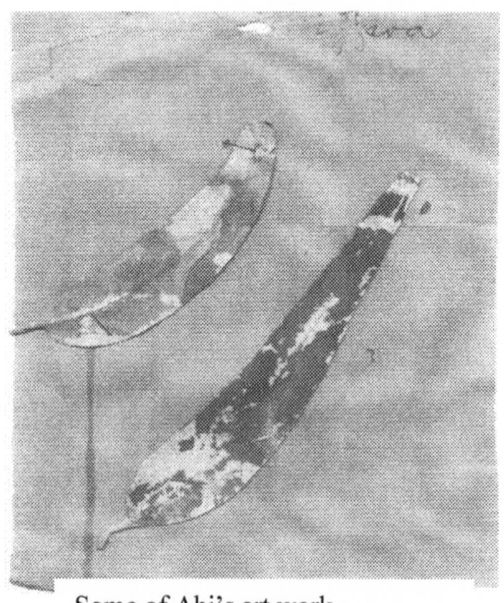

Some of Abi's art work

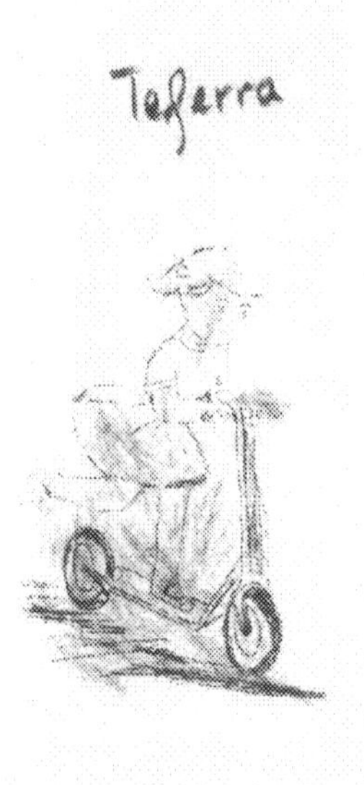

Some of Abi's art work

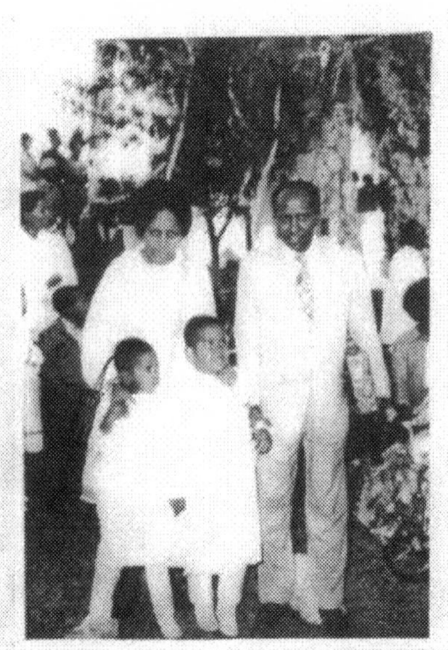

Abi with his brother and parents

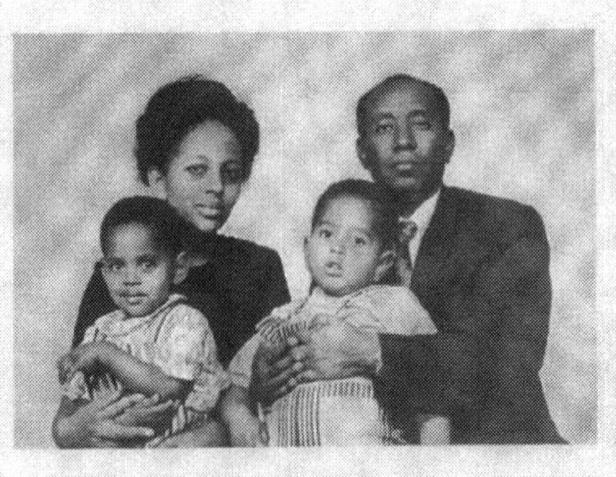

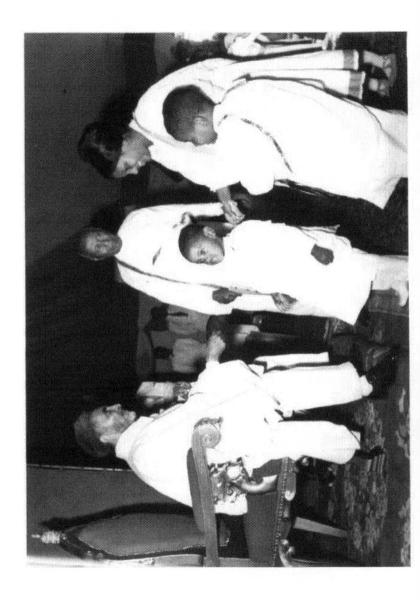

A picture at the palace - with the Emperor at Christmas

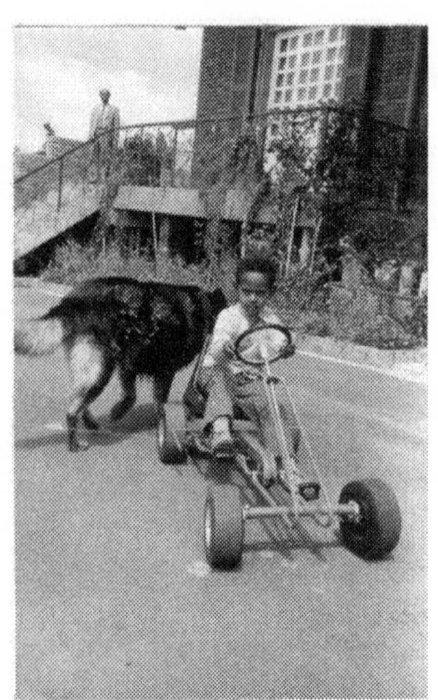

Abi with his father (in background)

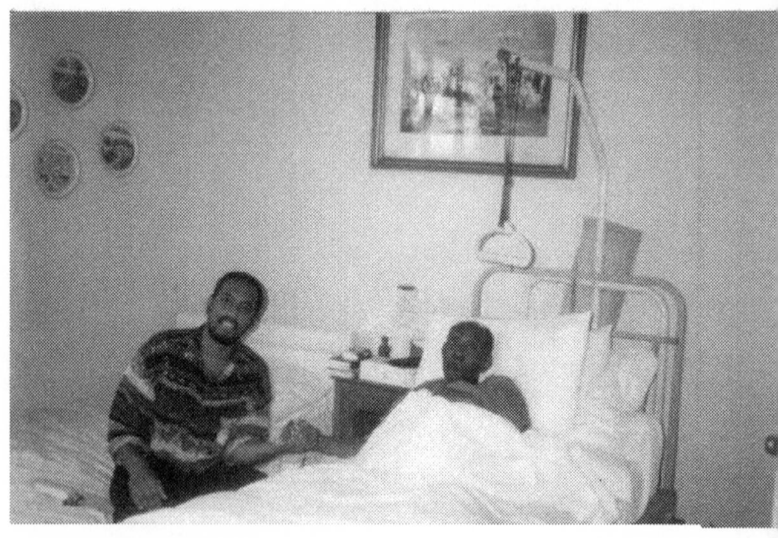

One of the last photos before fhis death: photo with his father

This period of instability and change had greatly affected both the boys. Our lives had changed drastically and both boys had wanted to understand why. However, the biggest change that affected Abi had been Hailegiorgis' imprisonment. His baby sister Memmenasha was just six months old and I had been nearly three months pregnant with Lelo. We realized how this memory of instability and uncertainty was embedded in Abi's mind much later on when as a young man he described to me how he understood the horrors of those times.

I myself had felt totally shattered by Hailegiorgis' imprisonment and I recall the morning after his arrest as having been very painful. Mammush and Abi had a habit of jumping into our bed every morning. As usual they both walked in to our bedroom to find half the bed empty and found me fully dressed having had difficulty sleeping that night. Abi had expressed his feeling openly and had demanded an explanation. I had then tried to explain the events that were taking place as accurately as one could and in a way that a child would understand. However, visitors who came to consol us would give alternative versions of the events. Stories like Hailegiorgis being abroad, or coming back soon, which were attempts to protect the boys from the situation, proved to be very confusing and increased their feelings of doubt and uncertainty. Abi, later on, described this time of his life as 'shattering'.

Imprisonment in those days required home support. Meals had to be carried to the prison three times a day. Clothes would be washed at home, and other basic necessities were provided from home. One day when both Abi's grandparents went to visit, and make deliveries for Hailegiorgis in prison, Abi spoke out on his and his brother's behalf, demanding for the same opportunity, saying, "otherwise tell the truth whether he is still around or not". When Hailegiorgis found out about what Abi had said, he was so concerned, that he immediately got special permission to see his two sons.

Workneh and Abi had started attending the English community school and initially they seemed reasonably happy there. Every morning I took them to school and on the way we would sing " He's got the whole world in His hand" and "Combya my Lord Combaya". We enjoyed these times we had together and on the surface, at least, the boys tried to make the best of the situation in which we found ourselves.

The birth of Lelo during this period gave us joy and worked as positive preoccupation for all of us. Meanwhile, we prayed, waited and hoped for the release of Hailegiorgis. In September 1975, on Ethiopian New Year's eve, some prisoners were released. Among them was a close friend of Hailegiorgis'. The fact that their father was not released at the same time had upset the boys a lot. However, Abi had heard optimistic prisoners' wives saying some more prisoners would be released for the feast of Meskel on 27th of September and this had created a false hope, which later proved to have been disappointing.

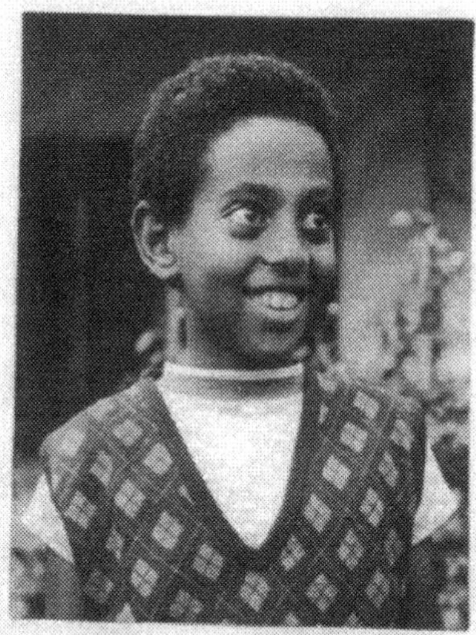

Pictures taken whilst Dad was in prison

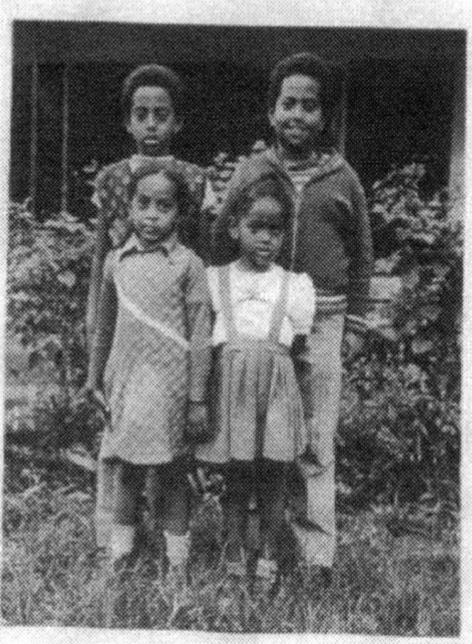

ሰባተኛ ፡ ቀን ፡ አድቬንቲስት ፡ ትምህርት ፡ ቤት ።

Seventh-day Adventist School

የተማሪ ፡ ማመልከቻ ።

STUDENT REPORT

የትምህርት ፡ ቤት ፡ ስም ፡ __________
Name of School

የተማሪው ፡ ስም ፡ __________
Name of Student

ዕድሜው ፡ __________
Age

የገባበት ፡ ቀን ፡ 3/7 _____ የወጣበት ፡ ቀን ፡ 27/73
Entered Withdrawn

ክፍሉ ፡ __________
Grade (Class)

ወደ ፡ ክፍል ፡ ተዛውሯል ፡ __________
Promoted to Grade (Class)

የትምህርት ፡ ዘመን ፡ 1973 ዓ.ም.
School Year

THE SANDFORD ENGLISH COMMUNITY SCHOOL
P. O. BOX 30056 MA
ADDIS ABABA

PREPARATORY DIVISION

REPORT FOR FIRST/~~SECOND/THIRD~~ TERM 1977

NAME Teffera Haile Ghiorghis CLASS P2/3.

Subject	COMMENTS
English	Teffera is reading well now and is beginning to write by himself.
Amharic	[illegible]
Maths.	Teffera works well. He answers well in oral work and written exercises reach a satisfactory standard. He has understood all the new work we have done.
Activities	Teffera enjoys all musical activities and sings well. He also joins in very enthusiastically in P.E.
General Comment	Teffera continues to make satisfactory progress. He is well behaved and keen to do well.

J. M. Brereton Class teacher

[signature] Headmaster C. A. German Division Head

Next Term commences on Jan. 17th '78

THE SANDFORD ENGLISH COMMUNITY SCHOOL
P.O. BOX 30056 MA

JUNIOR DIVISION
ADDIS ABABA MICHAELMAS TERM
School Year 19 78 19 79

Name: TEFERRA HAILE GIORGIS

CLASS: P3/3

SUBJECT	REMARKS	GRADE
English	Teferra's English is fairly good. He should try and pay attention in class and concentrate harder on his work.	C
Maths	Teferra's maths is also fairly good, if somewhat untidy at times. He must listen carefully.	C
Science		
Social Studies	Teferra shows a lively interest in this subject. He should try to make his work neater though.	C
Amharic	[illegible]	C-
Art	Teferra shows a good use of colour and a lively imagination.	B-
Physical Education	Teferra is a lively athlete and is a keen runner. Good	Not graded.

School Grading System: A - Excellent B - Good C = Fair, D-Pass, F - Fail

General Comment: Teferra tends to dream instead of work. At other times he is too concerned with the activities of other people. He tends to become overexcited. He must concentrate more.

Headmaster [signature] Class Teacher [signature]

Date 11 XII 78. Division Head [signature]

Next Term begins on [illegible] JANUARY 1979 Next term ends on [illegible] APRIL 1979

I had pointed out that nearly a year ago worse things had happened and sixty officials had been executed and the best we could do would be to pray that their father would come out in God's own time. Abi still did not accept his father would not be released until the disappointment of delivering meals at the prison on Meskel day. On returning home Abi's tears rolled down his face as he said' Meskel has been and gone and Ababaye never got released".

After the Meskel day incidence both boys started to demand that I should collect them form school. They had become fearful and insecure about my safety. True to their fears I was arrested and taken to prison in February 1976. Abi later told me that, though he hadpretended to be asleep, on the afternoon of my arrest, he had seen the soldiers with machine guns walking into his bedroom and had also heard them walk into his sisters bedroom. Abi had also witnessed my mother's arrest while he was at home having lunch with her. He later told me that on that day he decided that all the family would gradually be arrested and he, his brother and his sisters would end up on the street. Witnessing his grandmother's arrest had shattered him and it was yet another traumatic experience which left him feeling extremely insecure. The years also passed with the hope that each New Year would bring about our release from prison and each year the disappointment strengthened the feelings of uncertainty for the children.

The children had lived, for a short while, in the house that my husband and I built. After our imprisonment the house was confiscated and the children had to move twice. This had been very unsettling. Further instability came when the boys were withdrawn from Sandford School and sent to Seventh Day Adventist Boarding School. Abi understood and described all these events as "preparation to be orphaned". He feared that his parents would not come out alive and that life would never return to normal. During this period of his life, like children of his age, Abi enjoyed playing football with his brother, sisters and other children from the neighborhood. Some of the things Workneh remembers about his brother was that during the imprisonment of his mother and father he developed a great attachment to his grandmother who lived the other side of their house; she used to prepare him his favorite dishes of mixed salad and Ketffo (an Ethiopian dish made from spices minced meat). Workneh also remembers that Abi had enjoyed wrestling with him. Abi enjoyed board games and was particularly good at Chinese checkers. However,
at this time in Abi's life, his brother and sisters had noticed that Abi had become more withdrawn as he was constantly ill and experienced nightmares regularly. My mother took him often to receive holy water at the Orthodox church and this helped a great deal to reduce the frequency of the problem. Looking back now, we feel that these were

some of the first signs of Abi's depression even though at the time we just accepted it as Abi being Abi.

ሰባተኛ ፡ ቀን ፡ አድቬንቲስት ፡ ትምህርት ፡ ቤት።

Seventh-day Adventist SChool

የተማሪ ፡ ግሬድ ።

STUDENT REPORT

የትምህርት ፡ ቤት ፡ ስም ፡
Name of School

የተማሪው ፡ ስም ፡
Name of Student

ዕድሜ ፡
Age

የገባበት ፡ ቀን ፡ 2/74 የወጣበት ፡ ቀን ፡ 25/74
Entered Withdrawn

ክፍል ፡ 6ኛ
Grade (Class)

ወደ ፡ ክፍል ፡ ተዛወረ ፡
Promoted to Grade (Class)

የትምህርት ፡ ዘመን ፡ 1974 ዓ.ም.
School Year

ትምህርት ። SUBJECTS	1ኛ ሴሚ 1 Semester	2ኛ ሴሚ 2 Semester	መጨረሻ Final Gr.
መጽሐፍ ቅዱስ Bible	87	78	83
አማርኛ Amharic	67	57	62
እንግሊዝኛ English	89	91	90
ሒሳብ Arithmetic	83	73	78
ጂኦግራፊ Geography	76	75	76
ታሪክ History			
ሳይንስ Science	79	65	72
ሐይጂን Health & Safety			
ሥዕል Drawing			
የሙዚቃ ትምህርት Music			
የሰውነት ማጠንከሪያ ት. Physical Education			
ባልትና Homemaking	68	67	68
እርሻ Agriculture	75	54	65
	8/58	14/57	

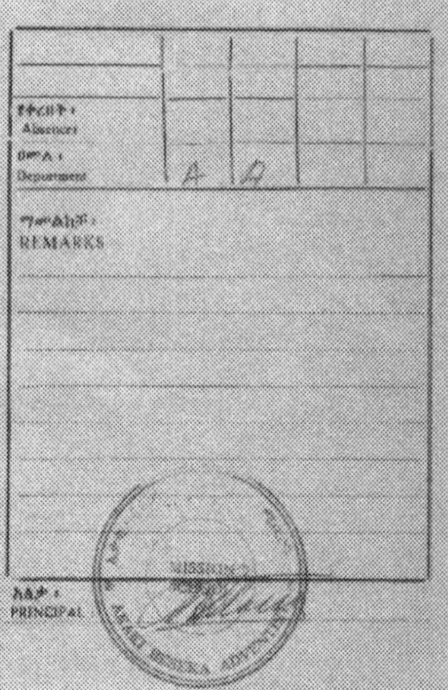

Absences				
Deportment	A	A		

REMARKS

PRINCIPAL

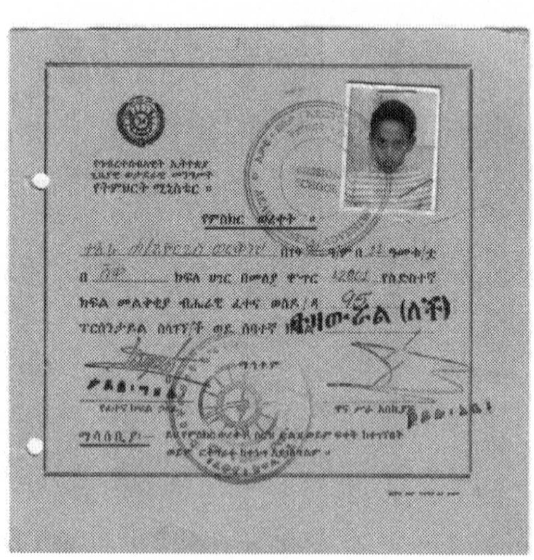

STUDENT GRADE REPORT

SEMESTER 1st Mid NAME TEFERA H/GIORGIS

SUBJECT	GRADE	REMARK
BIBLE	88	
AMHARIC	57	
ENGLISH	84	
MATHEMATICS	83	
GEOGRAPHY } SO. ST		
HISTORY	91	
BIOLOGY } SCIENCE		
CHEMISTRY	84	
PHYSICS		
HOME ECONOMICS	86	
TYPING		
WOOD WORK		
RANK	1/76	
CONDUCT		

Parents Signature

PRINCIPAL

6th Grade National Exam result, 1982

ሰባተኛ ፡ ቀን ፡ አድቬንቲስት ፡ ትምህርት ፡ ቤት ፡

Seventh-day Adventist School

STUDENT REPORT

Name of School [illegible] MISSION SCHOOL

Name of Student TEFERA H/GEORGIS

Age

Entered Sept.13/[illegible] Withdrawn Jul.1/[illegible]

Grade (Class) SEVEN

Promoted to Grade (Class) 8

School Year [illegible]

SUBJECTS	1st Semester	2nd Semester	Final Gr.
[illegible]	58	61	70
Bible	72	65	69
Amharic	91	93	92
English	–	–	–
Algebra	100	93	[illegible]
Geometry	–	–	–
Trigonometry	93	100	[illegible]
Geography	–	–	–
History	52	100	76
Science	–	–	–
Biology	–	–	–
Chemistry	–	–	–
Physics	–	–	–
Music	–	85	–
Physical Education	80	91	76
Domestic Science	–	–	–
Industrial Arts	–	–	–
Agriculture	[illegible]	[illegible]	[illegible]
Commercial			

Absences				
Deportment	A	A		
REMARKS				

PRINCIPAL [illegible]

ሰባተኛ ፡ ቀን ፡ አድቬንቲስት ፡ ትምህርት ፡ ቤት ፡

Seventh-day Adventist School

የተማሪ ፡ ማመልከቻ ፡

STUDENT REPORT

የትምህርት ፡ ቤቱ ፡ ስም ፡ A.A. School
Name of School

የተማሪው ፡ ስም ፡ TEFERA H/GIORGIS
Name of Student

ዕድሜው ፡
Age

የገባበት ፡ ቀን ፡ [illegible] የወጣበት ፡ ቀን ፡ [illegible]
Entered Withdrawn

ክፍል ፡ [illegible]
Grade (Class)

ወደ ፡ ክፍል ፡ ተዛወረ ፡
Promoted to Grade (Class)

የትምህርት ፡ ዘመን ፡ 1953/54
School Year

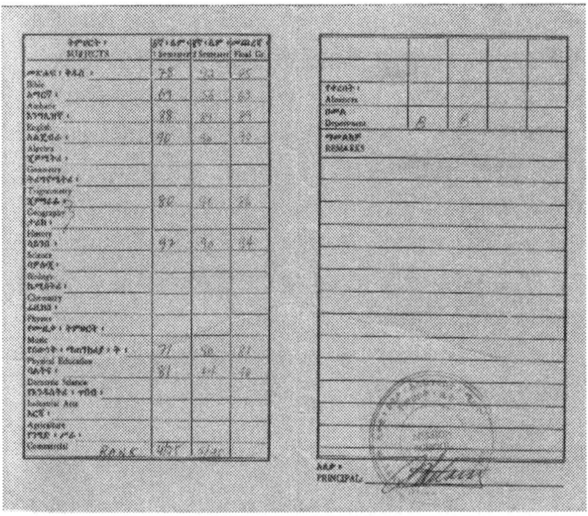

SUBJECTS | 1 Semester | 2 Semester | Final Gr.

Bible
Amharic
English
Algebra
Geometry
Trigonometry
Geography
History
Science
Biology
Chemistry
Physics
Music
Physical Education
Domestic Science
Industrial Arts
Agriculture
Commercial

Absences
Deportment
REMARKS
PRINCIPAL

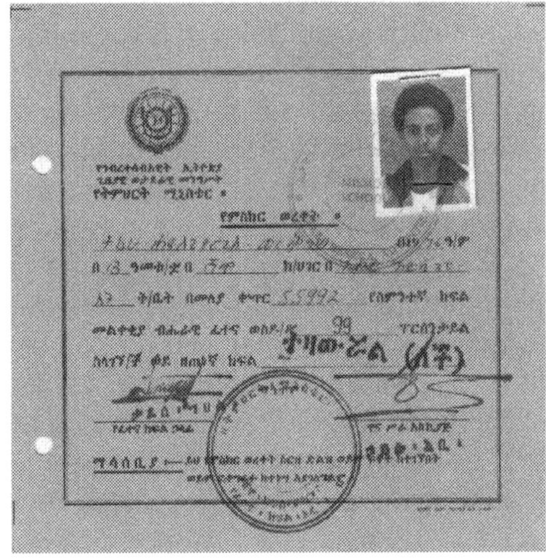

8th Grade National Exam result. 1984

God is good and I was released in February 1981 after five years of imprisonment and Hailegiorgis came out of prison soon afterwards, in September 1982, after eight and half years of imprisonment. It was a period of adjustment and happiness mixed. He used to repeatedly play the then popular ABBA record " I have a dream". It was much later after our release that Abi talked openly about the pain of the years during our imprisonment. Immediately after our release, though, Abi went through his own version of adjusting to life with parents, as all the other children did and he continued to do extremely well at school and to show us his keen and inquisitive mind which questioned everything from world politics to the Bible, Marxist philosophy and all kinds of socio-political issues. He was extremely politically aware and when I came out of prison we spent a lot of time discussing all these issues as he had questions about Marxism and Leninism. The cold war fascinated him and one of his comments on the East/West political situation was to describe Breznev and Regan as " the worst gangsters in the world". As a teenager he was a fearsome political debater and had a highly competitive character in sports and games.
He had a photographic mind and had a fascination for cars, aeroplanes and enjoyed remembering car registration numbers of all the people he knew.

During the enforced conscription in 1983, Abi, once again, felt insecure and as a teenager he understood better the threats of war and how this would affect his life. Abi saw this situation as another hurdle that he had to cross. With God's help and friends' support, scholarship and bursary were found to send both boys to the United Kingdom. Getting permission to leave the country was a miracle. Abi later described leaving Ethiopia as a "dilemma" because he felt torn between staying, enjoying his parents in a normal family life and fleeing from his country to save his life. He left. He had ended up choosing to save his life! In September 1984, the boys left for the United Kingdom and they were fortunate enough to be accompanied by their father. When I cried at the airport, Abi told me off saying "what would God say when you cry after trying and praying for us to be rescued from conscription?" Abi always had a way of saying the right thing at the right time!

Adjusting to life in England was difficult for Abi and the new English Public School environment was very different to what both boys had left behind. He had to quickly adapt from the cultures and disciplines of an Ethiopian Adventist boarding school to an English public school which could not be more different. The adjustment had been a stressful and daunting task for a boy of 13 years old. Abi found his school years difficult. His sisters recall him talking about being bullied at school. His brother remembers that Abi's peers resented his achievements and their recognition he received from the school for his numerous victories as a cross-country runner. This lead to relentless bullying using his colour, his personality and his foreign student status as an excuse for picking on him. As a result, Abi made very few close friends. The strength by which he resisted and responded to these bullies would have taken its toll and contributed to the mental health problems, which eventually caused his illness. Abi enjoyed socializing and spending quality time with his family. However, after his illness, being with people became very difficult for Abi and he would try and avoid social situations as much as possible, which in turn increased his sense of isolation.

Thankfully, it was not all doom and gloom both boys were able to carry out their studies and pass their GCE and A-Levels exams. Like most teenagers, Abi enjoyed music, he loved the cinema and his favourite actor in the eighties was Eddie Murphy. He loved listening to music by Alexander O'Neil, Barry White, Neway Debebe and ABBA. Abi was also an able sports man he was especially talented in athletics in long and middle distance running. He won medals for races in Cheltenham, the town where his school was located and the town where he stayed with family.

Family holidays were greatly enjoyed during my Master study at Manchester University 1986 – 1989. We spent holidays in France, Austria, Germany, Switzerland and Finland as well as Sweden, Norway and Denmark as well as holidays in the U.K. all of which were the happy days we as a family fondly remember. Whenever it was his turn to keep me carry my luggage he would tease me by saying, “Don’t pack heavy things which you cannot carry”.

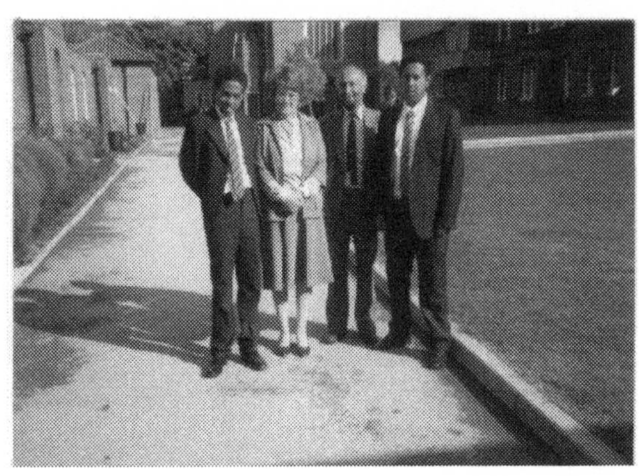

Abi at Dean Close School

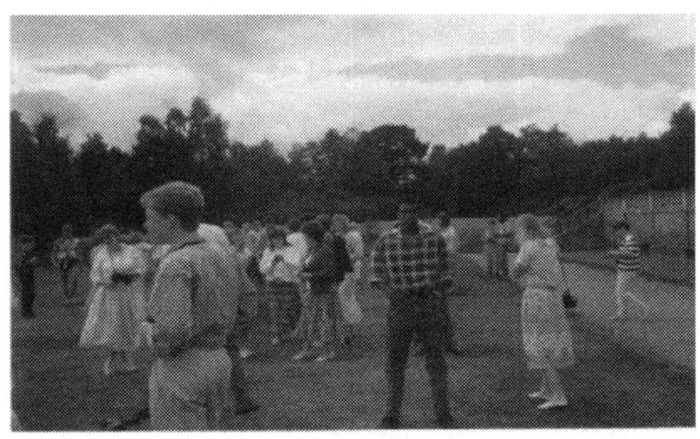

17-9-84

To Emmama,

Emmama, how are you? I am well except missing you. How is the family? How are Memmenasha and Pupy? Are they OK? Please greet them for me I understand their school term begins soon. Please tell them to do well at school. How is Yetot? Please greet her for me. How is Emaye? Greet her for me. Please greet Wossenu, Gizachew and Henok. Please give my greetings to the household and our relatives.

Let me share with you about our journey. After we left home we arrived in Rome, from Rome to Frankfurt, then from Frankfurt we arrived in London where we were met by Gash Dawit and Mary. We met Eteye Negat then Mary left from the airport. We traveled with the underground train to out hotel, which was reserved for us, at Kensington Court, in Bayswater. Then on Saturday Mary and Nigel came and took us shopping after which they left.

On Saturday we went to Bexhill to visit Miss Page. But we were told that she would be away until Wednesday. We spent the day there and returned to London. On Tuesday we went to Sussex University and returned to London. After that we went straight to Cheltenham where our school is. We stayed with Liz Scotland for 2 days then went to Dean Close School. Liz's daughters have sent their regards to Memmenasha and Pupy. They received us warmly and gave us a good time. Apart from that we are enjoying school.

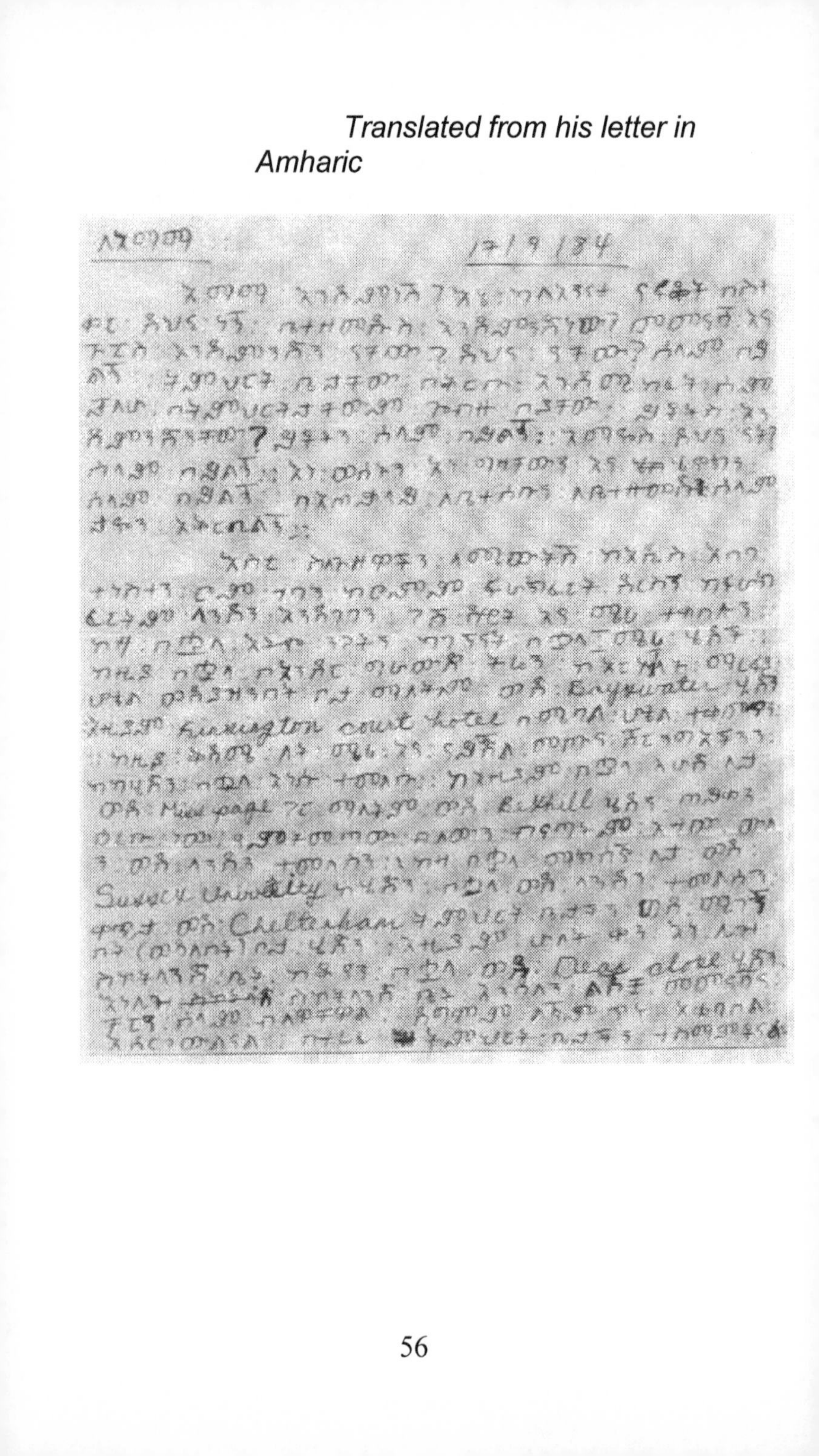

Translated from his letter in Amharic

ለእማማ 17/9/84

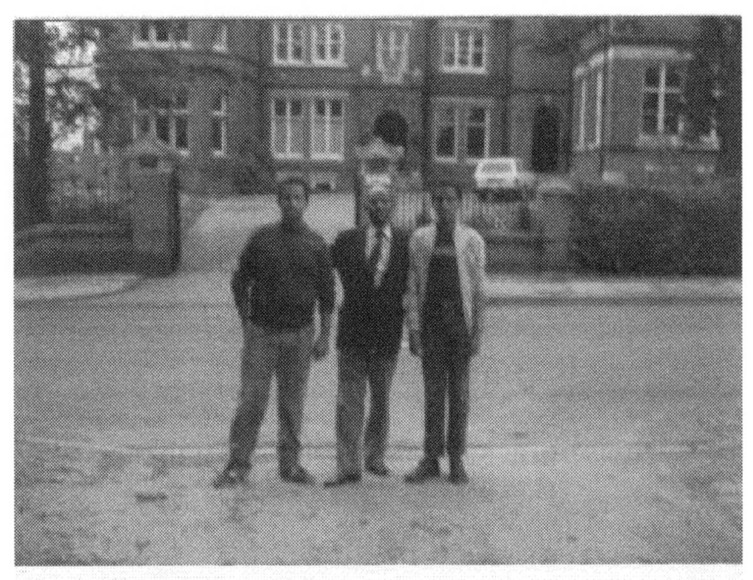

**Abi with his father and brother (above)
and with his uncle and brother (below)
at Dean Close School**

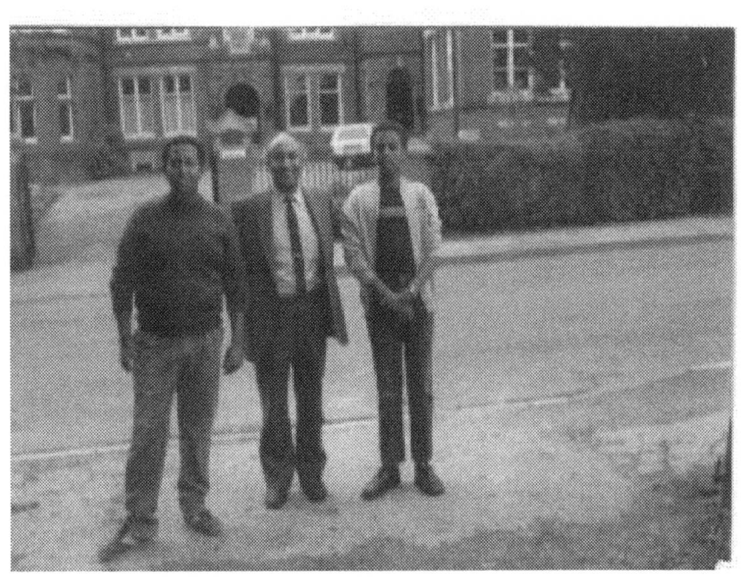

Name ..TEFERRA HAILE-GIORGIS.......................... HEADMASTER'S COMMENT

As everybody knows we are delighted to have Teferra in our midst and expect him, once he has mastered the language, to move on rapidly in his other classes. He has chosen to climb a big mountain, but I am confident that he can do it and we are all here with the ropes and other gear as well as the comradeship of encouragement. I love his smiling face and his enthusiasm for life.

Good bless you all at Christmas.

CERTS   Autumn Term 1984

:ties have been arranged to the following:

Welsh National Opera
C.B.S.O. (2 concerts)
English String Orchestra

tendance at up to two of these is without further charge for pupils
ceiving instrumental tuition. However, scholars who sign up for
e concerts in advance but fail to attend will, except in the case
illness, be charged.

ur son/daughter has taken the opportunity to attend ..0.. of these
ncerts.

Name .Tefera....Haile-Giorgis.   HOUSEMASTER'S REPORT

I am very encouraged by the content of these reports. Tefera is a very conscientious young man and if he can maintain this effort the future looks promising indeed. He is a most cheerful and popular member of Brook and his coming has brightened our lives considerably. He is even getting better at being in the right place at the right time!

Abi's first report (Two pages) at Dean Close School

October 1984

Emmama,

Emama how are you? I am fine except missing all of you. Ababa and Gash Dawit came to visit us.

I want to tell you something, you are the best parent letter writer amongst all Brook house student parents. When I wrote your comment on my half-term report you commented that it was pointed out that I am weak in English language. Thank God my English is improving. I now have 2 classes a week in English as a foreign language and 2 classes a week in French.

Otherwise please pass on my greetings to Yetot, to friends and family.

Abi.

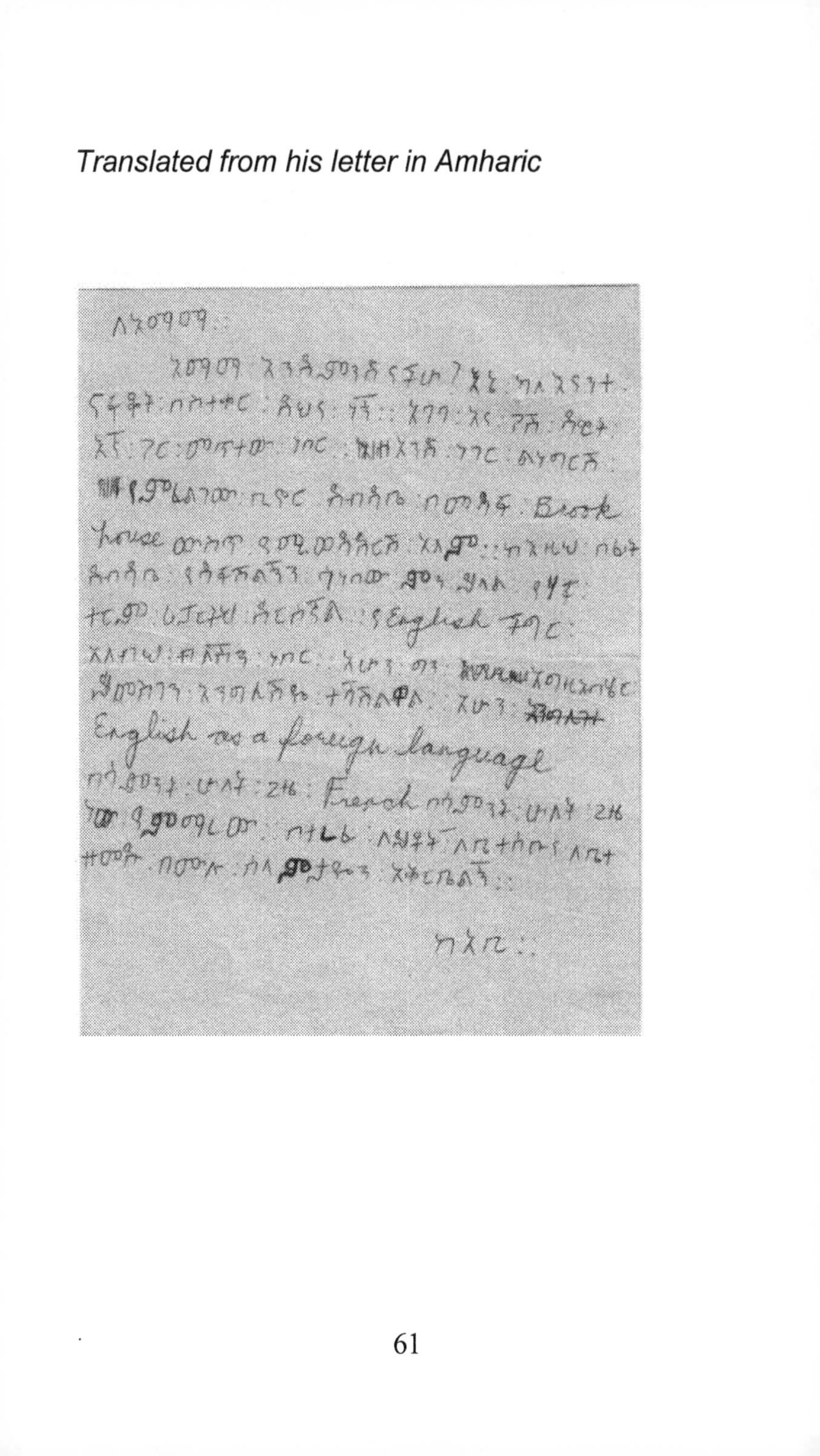

Translated from his letter in Amharic

When it came to time to going to university Abi struggled to choose a course. Though he had done science and math's for his A-levels he would have been much happier in arts or humanities. Though we suggested to him to go into humanities he was adamant to follow his father's area of work and opted for building studies. He opted for a subject which he felt would be useful if he ever went back to Ethiopia. He ended up going to Lancashire Polytechnic (now known as the University of Central Lancashire) and enrolled to do a HND in Building studies in order to be a quantity surveyor. His mathematics skills were strong enough to enable him to get into this field. However, his depression and his wish to remain isolated had already become apparent in his first year of study. It seemed that his first year of study was structured and this helped him to keep focused on his study. Looking at his assignment marks, we can see he had done well in his first year. In his second year (1990/91) it became apparent that his illness was taking over. His course supervisor pointed out that he had difficulty in working with his peers and as a team when group work assignment was given. His case supervisor also identified his depressive state and suggested temporary leave from classroom work. When I was visiting England during 1991, he told me he had something important to discuss with me. This was when he announced his mental illness to me. He had read books, analyzed and diagnosed himself. He told me that he suffered from depression and obsessive – compulsive behavior. The diagnosis was later confirmed by a psychiatrist after he admitted himself to Royal Preston ospital's, Avondale Unit, at the end of 1993.

Prior to his voluntary admittance into hospital, I had a memorable twelve hour conversation with him. He told me about the trauma he had suffered from the day of his father's arrest to the present time. He announced that he would never return home to Ethiopia since his illness began there. He declared that in 1974 it was a class persecution in the name of Marxism. In the new regime it is democracy through ethnic lines. He dreaded to think what would happen to us since he felt that his family was on the wrong side of politics again. He announced that if he would never return to Ethiopia for ten years and if he did go back it would be to remain in a monastery.

Abi had faith in God and throughout his illness he verbalized that only God would heal him. His religious stand, as a Christian, was uncompromising. He had a deep knowledge of the Bible which he had read from cover to cover. He always talked about the narrowness of the road to heaven and the excesses of the world. Even through his illness he was a thinker and enjoyed philosophizing about religion, politics and the anatomy of the brain in the context to his own illness. He Loved and admired John the Baptist and one of his desires was to be a teacher of the gospel on the streets of England. He often referred to what Christ said about John the Baptist in Matthew

Chapter 11 verse 11, "I tell you the truth, among those born of a women there has not risen anyone greater than John the Baptist; yet he who is least in the kingdom of heaven is greater than he". Teferra was a committed Christian he used to tell his brother and sisters, " I reconciled with Jesus at the age of 23 but you are lovers of life, admit it and repent of your sins"

Abi was socially conscious and had talked a great deal with me about helping the homeless. He had even gone to speak to churches to ask if they would help him help the homeless. Abi's faith in God has been a great comfort to us all. The pieces of papers we found after his death had written on them appeals for God to heal him. He had lost faith in the psychiatric treatment that he had received and felt that no one really understood the cause of his illness. In a number of meetings with the team of people who were responsible for his care, it became apparent to me, his carers did not know where Abi's case fitted. He had not seemed to fit into either "British black" mental health categories or other groups that they were exposed to. Abi has even walked out of such meetings feeling that it had been a waste of time and that the people around him would never understand his case. The drugs they gave him he described as "lifting him up when he was down, and putting him down when he was up". The side effect the drug had also caused him disorientation that led to his 24 hours detention in a London Police Station and appearing in court though he did not commit any crime and was acquitted. He has had several traumatic and victimization experiences due to his mental illness.

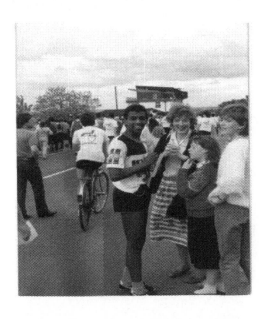

Sport achievement - Marathon award for Dean Close School and Cheltenham

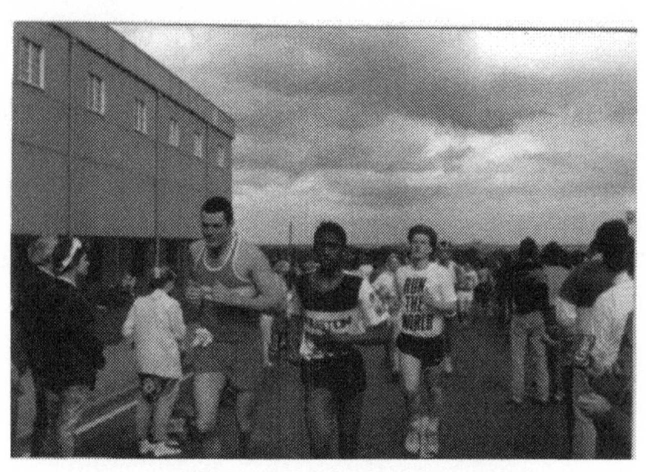

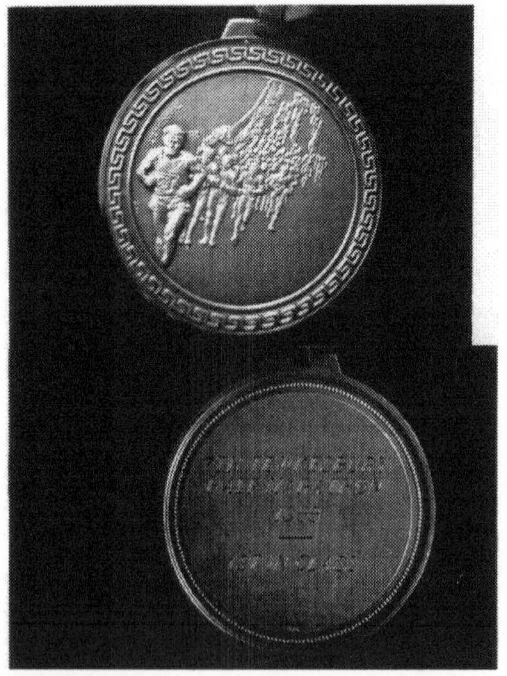

Medal for being 1st in the Marathon Run

Abi with families he lived within the U.K.

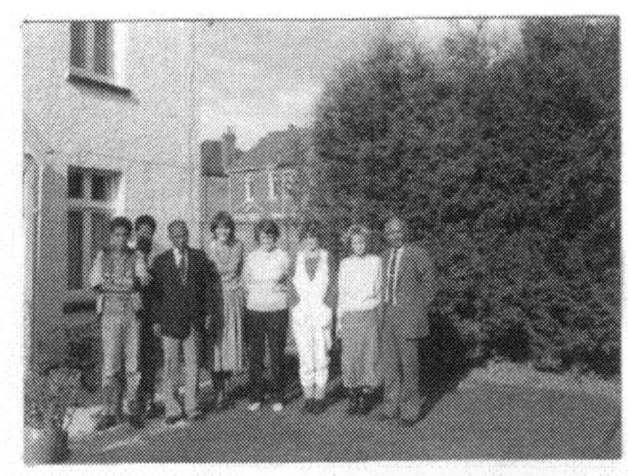

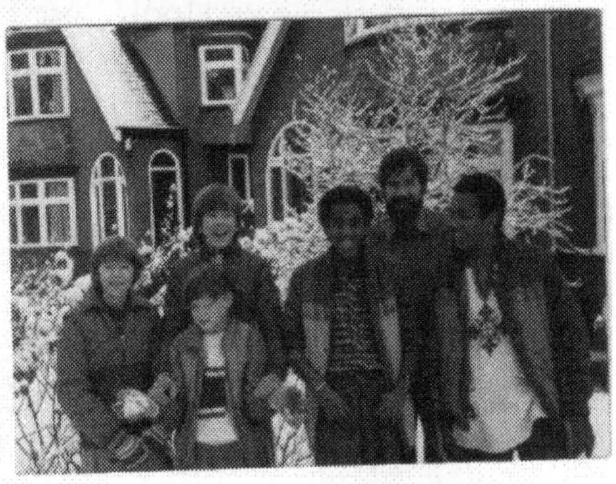

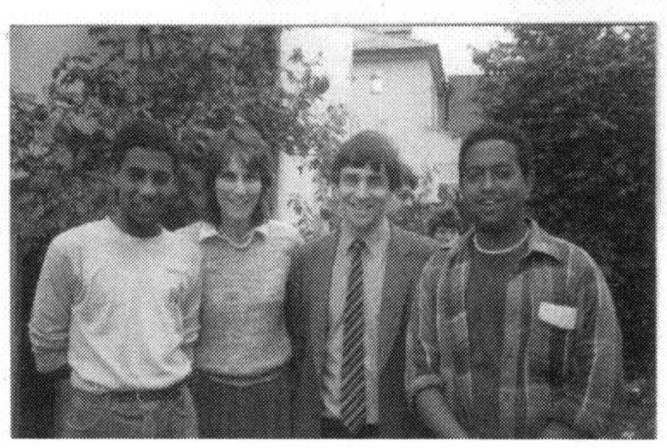

November 4th 1984, Cheltenham, England
To Emmama,

Emmama, how are you? We are well except missing you. I am sorry I have not written for a long time. I have been very busy.

We went to Mary's family for half-term. It was an enjoyable half – term. We visited Humber Bridge. Since they live close to the sea we also saw North Sea. Nigel and Mary bought us sport bicycles and instructed us as to how we should cycle in the town. During the holidays we can cycle. Nigel and Mary send their regards to you and the family.

We have received our half term exam results my marks are as follows. When you read my results S stands for satisfactory.

Subject	**Effort**	**Achievement**
English	S	C
French	S^+	B
Chemistry	S	C
Physics	S	A
Biology	S	C
Art	S^+	B^+
History	S	C
Geography	S	B
Maths	S	A

Otherwise please give my regards to the family. Please tell Memmenasha and Pupy that the reason why I have not written it because I am short of time. I hope to write to them soon. Good bye.

Abi

Translated from his letter in Amharic

November the 4th 1984,
CHELTENHAM,
ENGLAND.

ለእማማዬ::

... half-term ... half-term ... Humber bridge ... North sea ...

... half term ... Satisfactory ...

Subject	Effort	Achievement
English	S	C
French	S+	B
Chemistry	S	C
Physics	S	A
Biology	S	C
Art	S+	B+
History	S	C
Geography	S	B
Maths	S	A

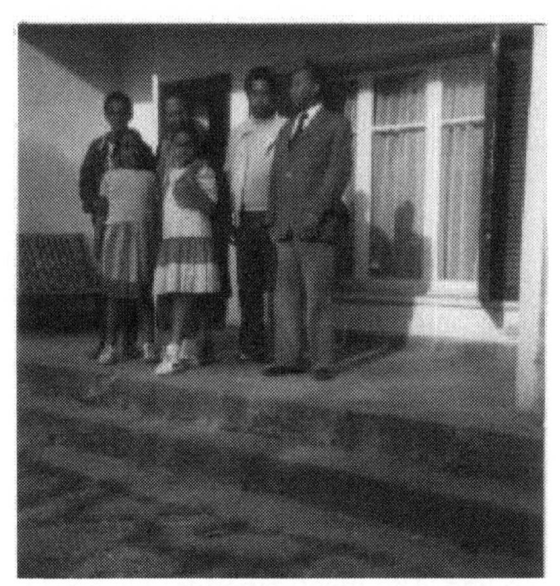

Abi with family as a group

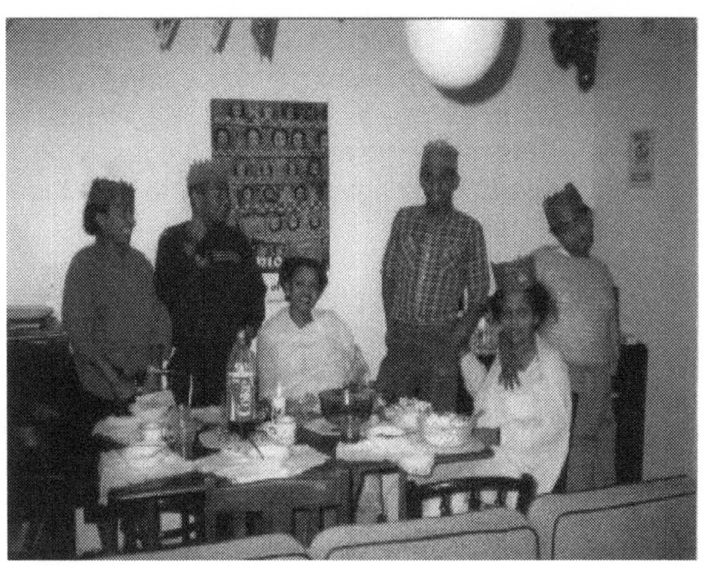

Summer 1987

Ababba,

Ababba, how are you? I am OK, thank God, except missing you and thinking about you. I am sure you will forgive me for not writing to you for so long. I have been very busy.

Having passed 3 “O” levels I started “A” level Maths course. When I complete 2 or 3 “O” levels I will start economics “a” level course. The most important thing is to study seriously.

At present I have started my holiday. I am busy studying to retake Physics and English language exams. I am staying with Nigel and Liz. They have moved to a new house which still needs to be finished. We try to help them in our free time.

Otherwise please pass on my greetings to Yetot, to Emaye, to Emamma and other members of family.

Abi

ለአባባ::

አባባ፡ እንደምን፡ አለህ? እኔ፡ ካላንተ፡ ሀሳብ የ፡ ላፍቅኝ፡ በስተቀር፡ እግዚአብሄር፡ ይመስገን፡ ደህና፡ ነኝ:: እስካሁን፡ ድረስ፡ ያልፃፍኩላህ፡ ስራ፡ ስለበዛብኝ፡ ነበር፡ እንድትገነዘብ፡ ይቅርታ፡ እንድ ታደርግልኝ፡ እጠይቅሃለሁ::

እኔ፡ ሶስት፡ O'level ፈተናዬ፡ Malta A'level ጀምሬያለሁ:: ሁለቱ፡ መጀመሪያ፡ ሶስት፡ O'level ከወሰድኩኝ፡ ሌላ፡ ሁለተኛውን፡ A'level (Economics) መማሬ፡ እጀምራለሁ:: ከEconomics ጋር፡ ሌላ፡ 'AO' level Business studies ሳልሰራ፡ አይቀርም:: ቀናው፡ ነገር፡ በርትቼ፡ መማሬ፡ ነው::

አሁን፡ እኔ፡ እረፍት፡ ላይ፡ ነኝ፡ ያለሁት:: አሁን፡ ለPhysics እና፡ English language retake በመማር፡ ላይ፡ ነኝ፡ ያለሁት:: እና፡ Nigel ሰፈር፡ ለመጠየቅ፡ አሌክስ፡ በወቅቱ፡ ወደ፡ ገብተናል፡ ታምሩ፡ ግን፡ አለብኝ፡ ስለዚህ፡ በትርፍ፡ ጊዜ፡ ያኔ፡ ተጫውተን፡ እንቀራለን

[illegible]፡ ለአጎቴ፡ ለአክስቴ

እና፡ ለሁሉም፡ [illegible]፡ ሰላም፡ በልልኝ:: ከተወዳጅ

Translated from his letter in Amharic

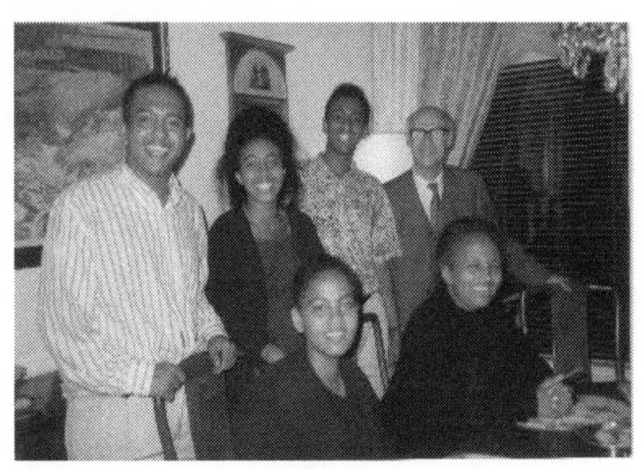

Holidays

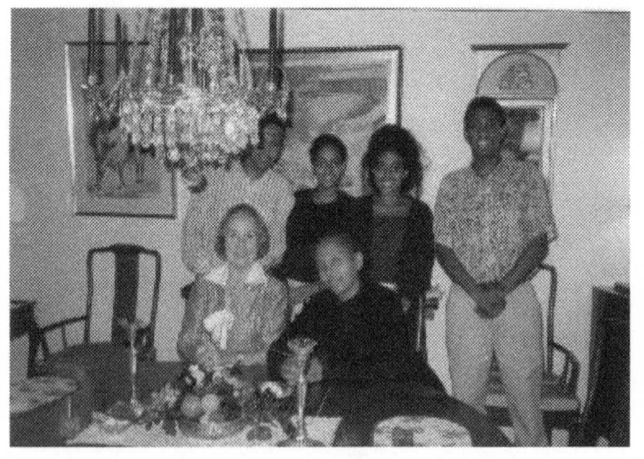

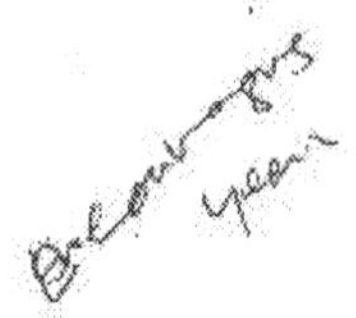

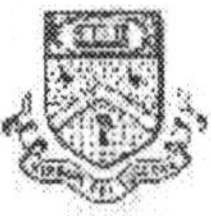

DEAN CLOSE SCHOOL

SCHOOL REPORT FOR SPRING TERM 1989

Name ...TEFERRA HAILE-GIORGIS

Age ..18.8..   Form ...U VI...

Next term : Boarders return Tuesday, 18th April.
Day Scholars report in by 8.30 next morning.

No formal Health Certificate is required but Parents or Guardians are responsible for ensuring that their children are free from infection when returning to School. Any case of doubt should be referred to the School Medical Officer before a Scholar's return.

Parents are reminded that a full term's notice must be given if a Scholar is leaving. Otherwise they will be liable for an additional term's fees.

Last Spring Term report before 'A' level (9 pages) Exam

SUBJECT Liberal Studies

Name Teferra Haile-Giorgis   Form ...U6...   Set ....

Grade (before exams) ....   No. in Set ....

He has often been willing to state an unusual point of view, and is a valuable and friendly member of the group.

O.G.H. Young

SUBJECT Economics

Name Teferra Haile-Giorgis Form Upper VI Set EC

Grade (before exams) .... No. in Set 7

He has made great strides in getting to grips with this subject and is within striking distance of success. He needs to maintain his efforts throughout. Colin Tinke.

Name Teferra Haile-Giorgis HOUSEMASTER'S REPORT

Teferra is coming to the awkward stage in his school career where he is beginning to outgrow the constraints and restrictions of the school system. He must work hard to stay within the bounds expected of him because though we may bend the rules we cannot change them just for one.

In class he is clearly working flat out but must try to channel this effort into slightly more productive directions. Quality as well as quantity of work is paramount.

In the House Teferra is usually good value and was especially noteable in the House Cross Country!

Richard Rignell

SUBJECT Mathematics......

Name Teferra Haile-Giorgis... Form U6......... Set 4...

Grade (before exams) .... No. in Set 3......

Teferra has continued to put a great deal of effort and enthusiasm into his maths this term. His trial exams were encouraging and showed promise, and he has built on it over the past weeks. Over the holidays he must try and learn as much as he can, and consolidate his understanding by doing plenty of A level questions.

Rachel Knight

SUBJECT ECONOMICS............

Name HAILE-GIORGIS, TEFERRA.... Form U6.......... Set ....

Grade (before exams) .... No. in Set 1.......

Teferra has made quite good progress this term, much more than I would have thought possible. He has got some way to go yet and the next three months must consist of unremitting work.

[illegible]

SUBJECT Economics......

Name Teferra Haile-Giorgis Form Upper VI. Set EC

Grade (before exams) .... No. in Set ...7.....

If anybody deserves success for lifting oneself out of a position of near hoplessness, then the award must surely go to this student. I very much hope this will be the case

Zedhie Turk

Name ..Teferra....Haile-Giorgis. HOUSEMASTER'S REPORT

Teferra has improved considerably as the year has progressed in many aspects of his life at Dean Close School. He is much more reliable and trusting that we are working for his own future and success. Obviously progress must be maintained - holiday reading is always a good starting point.

He has been much better in the House generally and his athletic ability much appreciated. He is to be congratulated on his being a member of the record breaking 4 x 400m relay team.

[signature]

Name TEFERRA HAILE-GIORGIS .... **HEADMASTER'S COMMENT**

Well done, Teferra. So many people are speaking in a praising voice of you and I am proud to note that.

I am sure he will listen wisely to Mr. Ryall's perceptive report and all of us are glad to note the most satisfactory offers which should be within Teferra's compass. All of us are prayerfully on the sidelines hoping for success and wish Teferra a very happy holiday accomplishing much by a disciplined revision programme.

Cal

May
1989

To Emmama,
Emmama, how are you? Thanks God, I am well except missing you. We are very happy to hear that Ababa is coming. We are awaiting for him. Thank you for sending me £5. My “A” level dates are as follows:

7th of June MATHEMATICS
PAPER 1
14th of June MATHEMATICS
PAPER 2
15th of June ECONOMICS
PAPER 2
20th of June ECONOMICS
PAPER 2
20th of June ECONOMICS
PAPER 3

I am writing a short letter because I am very busy. Until it is God’s will for us to meet again. Goodbye.

From your loving son
Teferra Hailegiorgis

Translated from his letter in Amharic

ለእማማ፡

[illegible] £5 [illegible] A' level date [illegible]

7th of June MATHEMATICS PAPER 1
14th of June MATHEMATICS PAPER 2
15th of June ECONOMICS PAPER 1
20th of June ECONOMICS PAPER 2
20th of June ECONOMICS PAPER 3

[illegible]

[illegible]

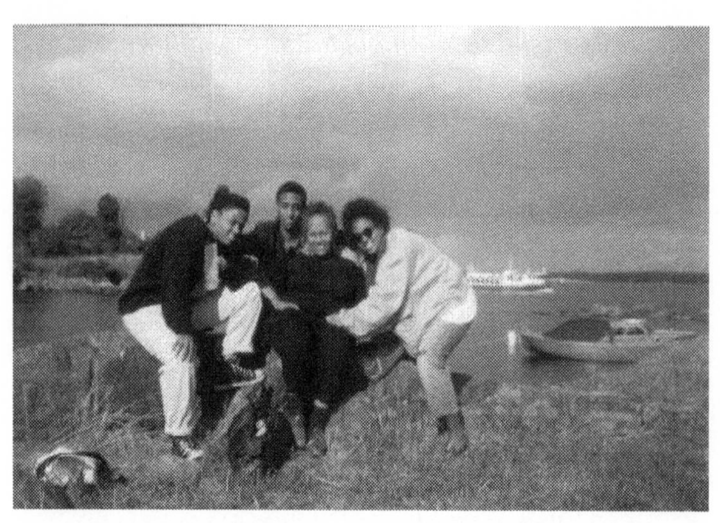

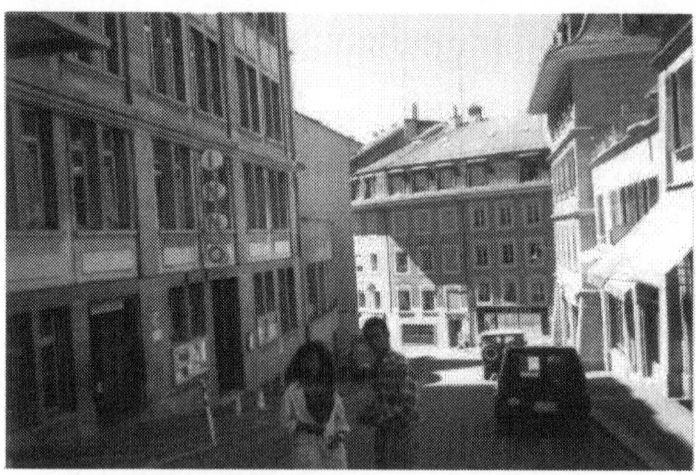

Holidays during mother's years in the UK (1986-89) with children: visit to Paris, Switzerland/Lausanne, Frankfurt/Cologne, Helsinki, Vienna, etc.

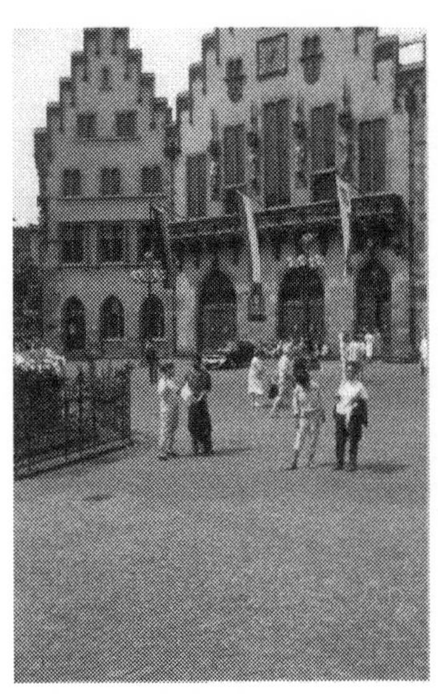

Holidays

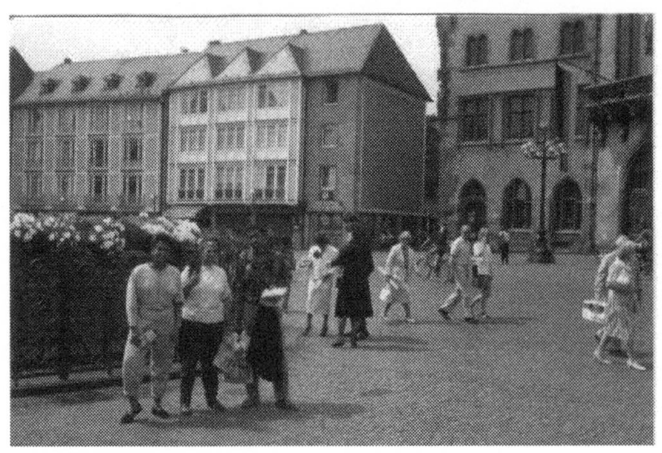

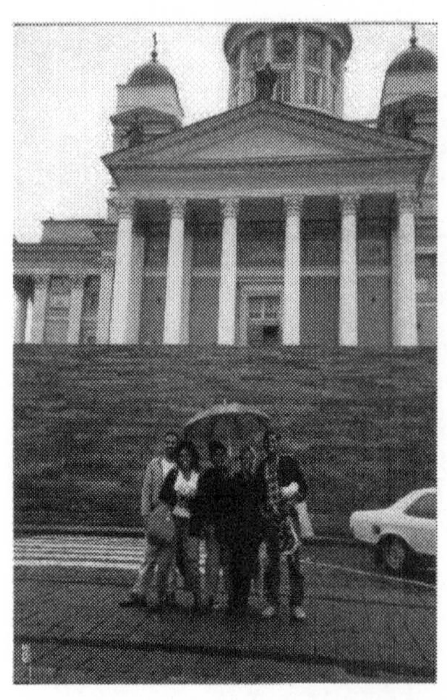

Holidays

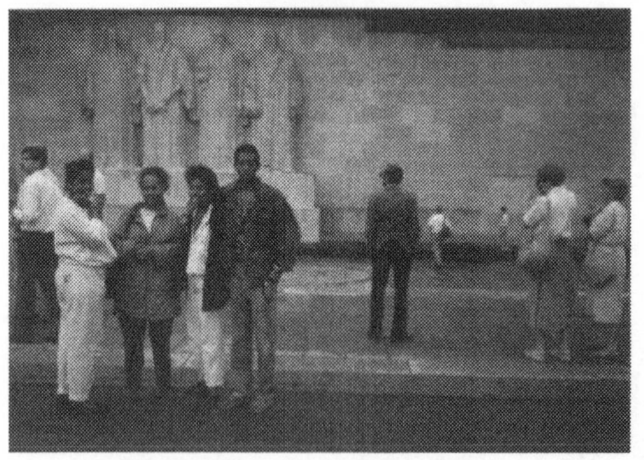

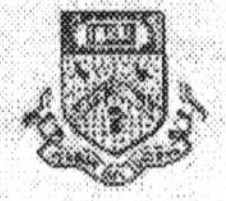

DEAN CLOSE SCHOOL

SCHOOL REPORT FOR SUMMER TERM 1989

Name ....Teferra....Haile-Giorgis..........

Age ....17.7....... Form ....UVI.......

Next term : Boarders return Monday, 4th September.
Day Scholars report in by 8.30 next morning.

No formal Health Certificate is required but Parents or Guardians are responsible for ensuring that their children are free from infection when returning to School. Any case of doubt should be referred to the School Medical Officer before a Scholar's return.

Parents are reminded that a full term's notice must be given if a Scholar is leaving. Otherwise they will be liable for an additional term's fees.

SUBJECT .Chaplain's name

Name Teferra Haile-Giorgis Form .....U6...... Set .....

Grade (before exams) .... No. in Set ....

" Come near to God and he will come near to you."

James 4.8

SUBJECT Mathematics.....

Name Teferra Haile-Giorgis.. Form U6.......... Set 4...

Grade (before exams) .... No. in Set 3.......

Teferra has worked hard this year with a good deal of enthusiasm, and deserves success in his A level.

I wish him all the best for the future.

Rachel Knight

SUBJECT ...Economics.....................

Name ...HAILE-GIORGIS,..TEFERRA. Form ....U6........ Set .....

Grade (before exams) .... No. in Set ...7.....

Teferra has completed an admirable amount of work in this subject and if anyone deserves to pass, he does. He has found the multiple choice difficult going but he should cope reasonably easily. Teferra has been pleasant at all times and I have enjoyed teaching him.

[illegible]

SUBJECT Economics.....

Name Teferra Haile-Giorgis Form Upper VI Set EC

Grade (before exams) .... No. in Set ....7....

He has made great strides in getting to grips with this subject and is within striking distance of success. He needs to maintain his efforts throughout. Cedric Tink.

TEFERRA HAILE-GIORGIS
Name .... HEADMASTER'S COMMENT

All of this is most commendable and I have been glad to find that Teferra feels the papers have been satisfactory. I certainly wish him all the very best for his University career and I am confident that he will go forward from strength to strength.

It has been lovely to have both the boys in the School and to have the acquaintance of the family. God's richest blessing on all of you and start off by having a lovely holiday.

CG

Summer 1989

To Ababba,

How are you? Thank God, I am well except missing you. I have now taken my 'A' level exams and started my holiday. For 2 weeks we were in Finland. It was not only a good holiday but also educational. Now I am awaiting for my exam results.

How are you and your health? Caroline wrote and told me that she enjoyed her visit in Ethiopia and her stay with you.

Otherwise please greet Yetot, Emaye and other members of the family. Until God reunites us in full health, good bye.

Translated from his letter in Amharic

ለአባባ፡

አባባ እንደምን [illegible] ነህ? እኔ [illegible] ናፍቆት
በስተቀር፡ እግዚአብሄር ይመስገን፡ ደህና ነኝ፡፡ አሁን፡
"A" level [illegible]
[illegible]
[illegible]
አሁን፡ ውጤቴን፡ በመጠባበቅ፡ ላይ፡ ነው ያለሁት፡፡
[illegible] ነህ? ።
Caroline [illegible]
[illegible]
[illegible]
[illegible]

[illegible]

[illegible]

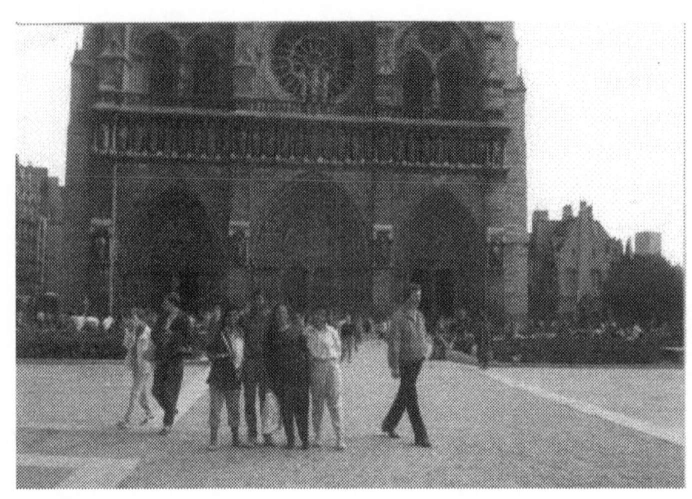

Holidays

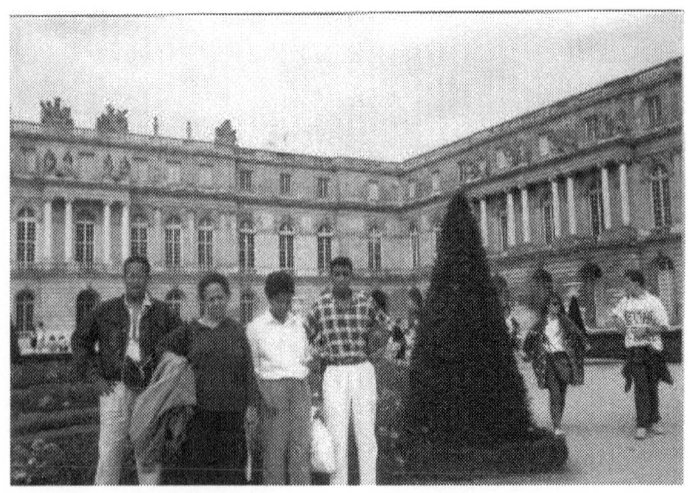

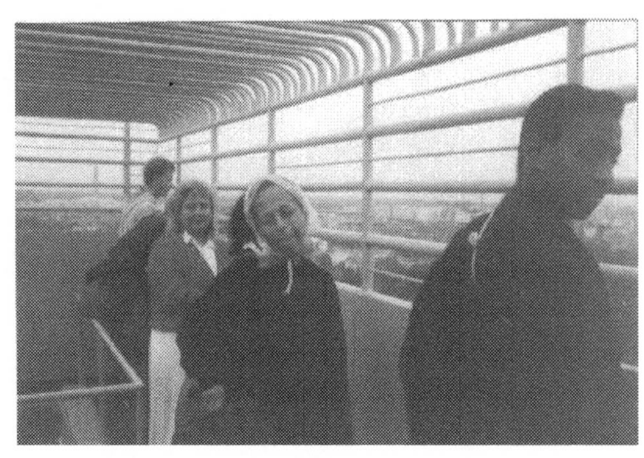

Holidays

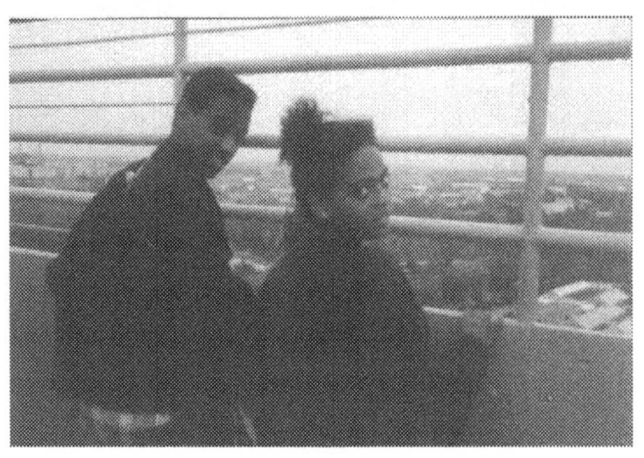

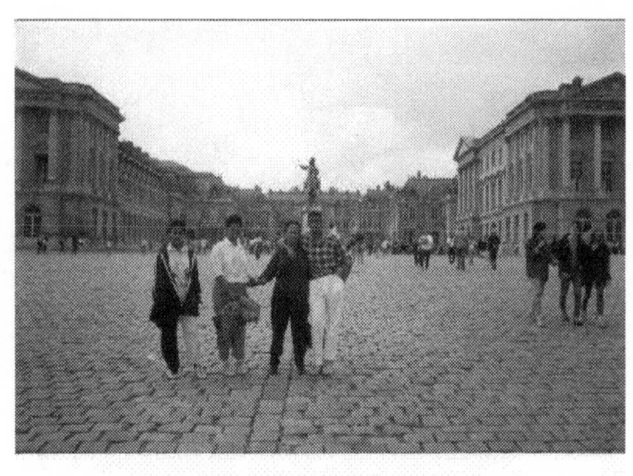

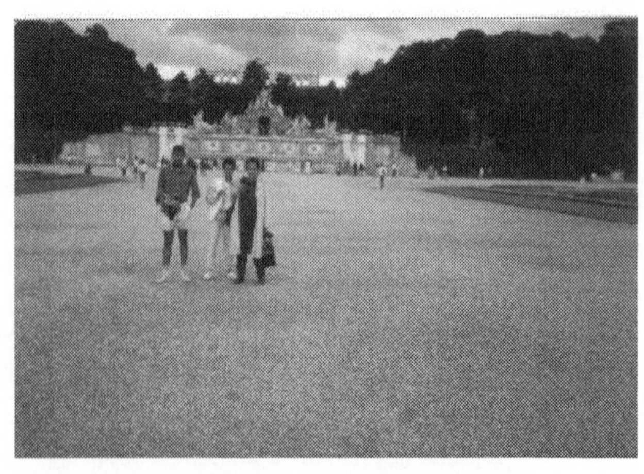

October, 1989

To Ababba, and Emmama,

How are you? I am well, thank God, except missing you I am acclimatized to everything; the course and, the environment are all good. Thank you for your letter and, Ababba, thank you for the book you sent me. It will be useful in the future.

I have completed my settlement programme: I have acquired one year visa, thank God, what is remaining is only the police registration.

I hope you are well and OK your end. Please pass on my regards to everybody. Until God reunites us in good health and peace good bye.

Teferra Hailegiorgis

Translated from a letter his Amharic

ለአባባና ለእማማ::

ከአገሬ፡ ናፋቂ፡ በስተቀር፡

እንደምን፡ አላችሁልኝ ደ/ እግዚአብሄር፡
ይመስገን ደህና ነኝ ሁሉም ነገር ተስማምቶኛል::
ትምህርቱም እንግሊዘኛውም ጥሩ ነው:: እናንተም ደስ ስ
ስለፃፋችሁልኝ አጋም መልሱ ስላላከልኝ በጣም
አመሰግናለሁ:: መልሱ ለመክፈት በጣም ያስቸግረኝ
ነው:: የእኔ Settlement programme
እስካሁን ተመዝግቤ የ እንዳ፡ አመት ፎቶ ቪዛ (VISA)
አላገኘሁም፡ ግን፡ አሁን፡ የሚቀረኝ፡ ፖሊስ Registration
ብቻ ነው:: ስለዚህ እግዚአብሄር ይመስገን::
በተረፈ እናንተም እንድትከባከቡኝ
ደህና፡ እንድትሆኑልኝ ተስፋ፡ አለኝ:: ሁላችሁም ሰላም
በሉልኝ:: እግዚአብሄር በሰላም፡ በጤና፡ እስከሚያገናኘን፡
ድረስ፡ ደህና ሁኑ::

ከልጃችሁ ከተስፋዬ፡ ሀይለጊዮርጊስ::

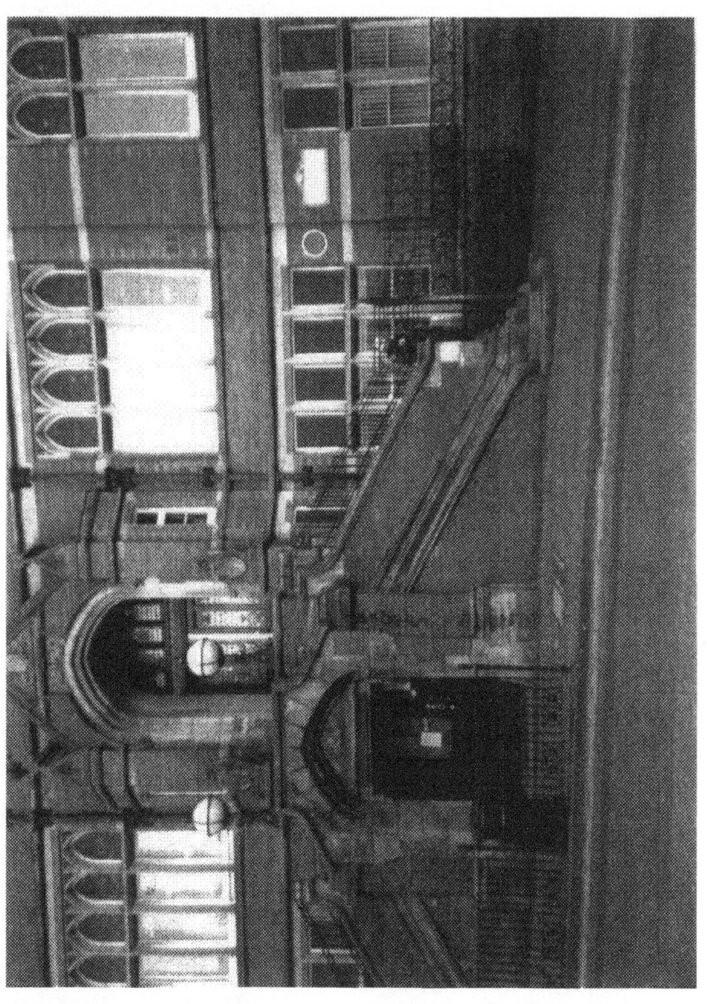

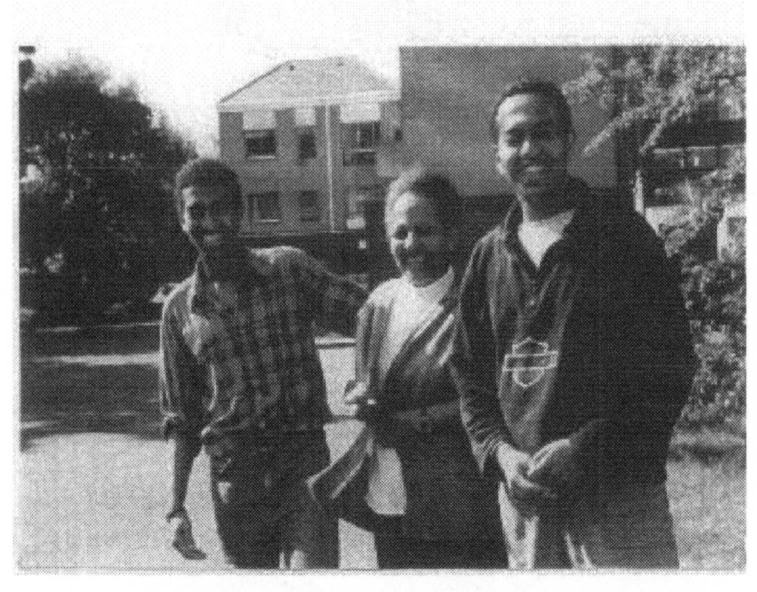

Abi with mother and brother

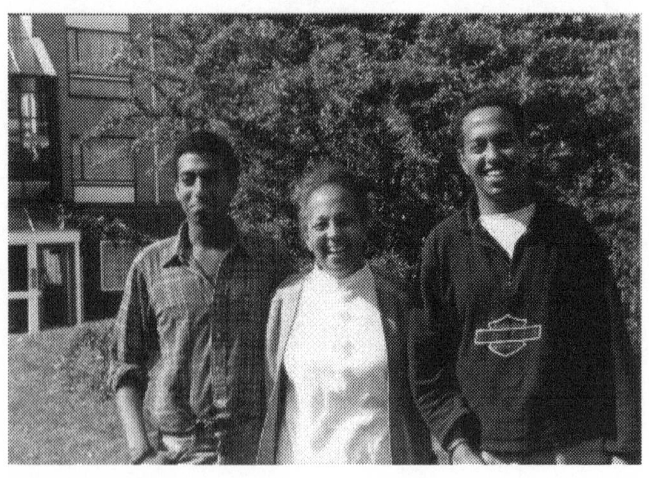

Abi with his brother

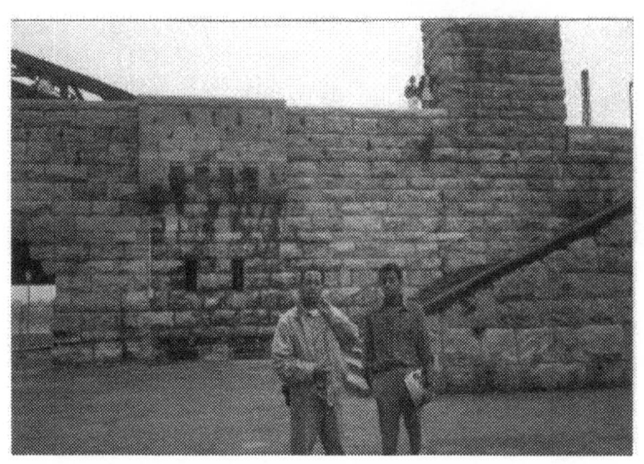

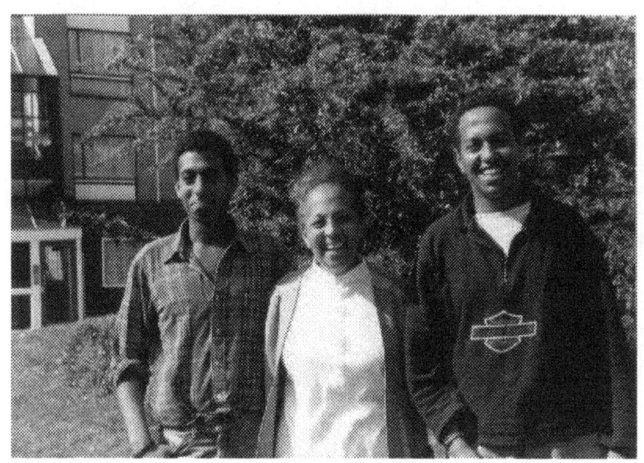

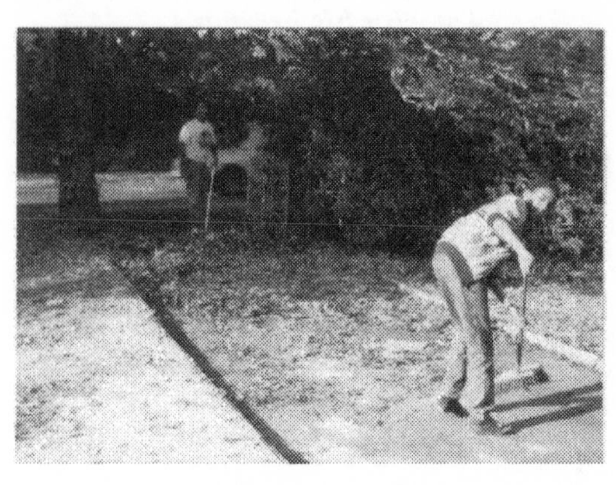

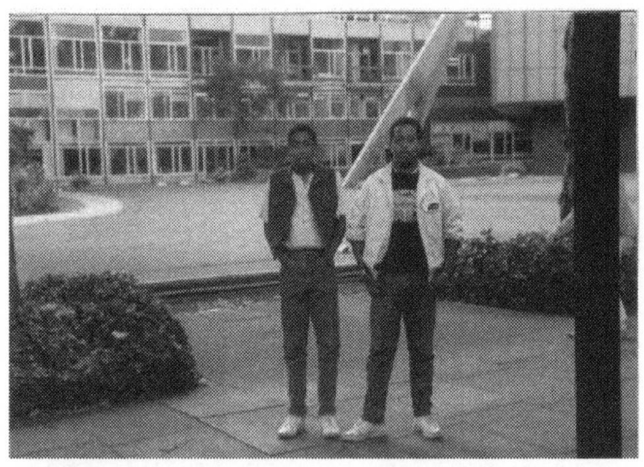

***Abi with his brother at the Commonwealth Trust* - 1985**

The last two years of Abi's life were very difficult for him. His illness seemed to have taken control and he would verbalise his wish to take his own life. He would also ask questions as to how God viewed the taking of one's own life. Less than a year before his death he had had an accident, which he told us, was a side effect of the drugs he was taking. When getting up from a toilet seat he lost control of his limbs, he fell and burnt his ear against the central heating pipes. Also as a result of this incident he developed a neurological problem in his left leg which made him limp. It seemed to us that Abi was giving up hope because, as a runner, loosing the proper use of his legs would have had a significant effect on him. At the time of the accident the doctors had wondered if it was a suicidal attempt, but later on confirmed that it was not, though he was re-hospitalized. In the last months before his death it was Abi's wish and only desire to return back to his flat in Preston. He went through at least two Tribunals to prove that he was well enough not to be kept in section and in hospital. He challenged the authority and the claim of efficacy of the mental health system, even as far as to writing to ministers in the Houses of Parliament. While in hospital he was well liked by the patient and nurses and would joke and make other patients laugh. He had created friendships within the hospital.

When he visited his father for the last time, before both died, and before Hailegiorgis returned home, Abi requested me to arrange a group discussion with his psychiatrist and others who dealt with him.

When this group discussion session was arranged in my presence one of the psychiatrist described his case as not fitting “into a British Black, or a British White” mental health problems. He did not know how to categorize him or classify him. Abi walked out of that session. Before closing the door he said to me “you are wasting your time, Emmama, these people are dummies. I have repeatedly told you that they do not understand my case. I think that if I ever get healed I will help other victims like myself. It would only be someone like me who has been through such illness that can help those in similar circumstances”. This was his last word that his family has taken as his appeal to help others who are victimized like himself. This last statement has also inspired his family to consider his appeal as wishing to help others in similar circumstances.

On the afternoon of Friday the 20th September 1996, Abi was found at the bottom of the 15 storey Guildhall building in Preston town center. He died at 3:50pm that afternoon as a result of multiple injuries which were the result of his jump from the top of the building. Abi had left no note to say goodbye or to explain the thinking which made him make this final decision. Instead in his pocket was found £40 pounds and a note which read ‘for the poor’. His death had been devastating to all of us and our grief had been intensified by the fact that he died

Abi with his father and brother

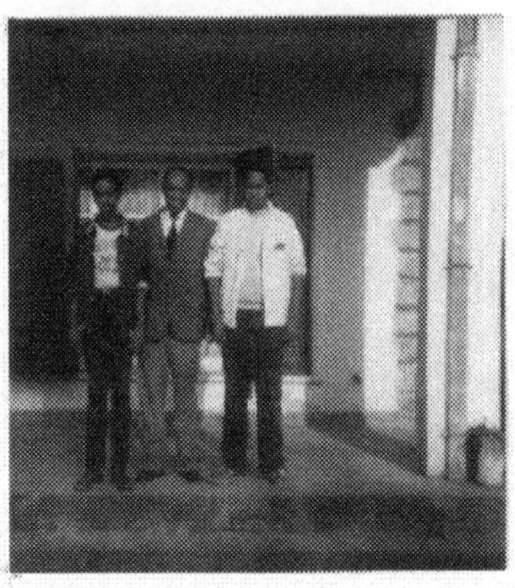

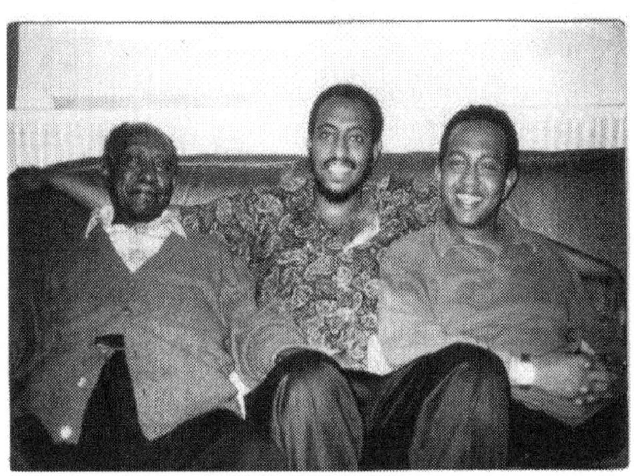

Spring/Summer 1994 - the Trios (half of the family)

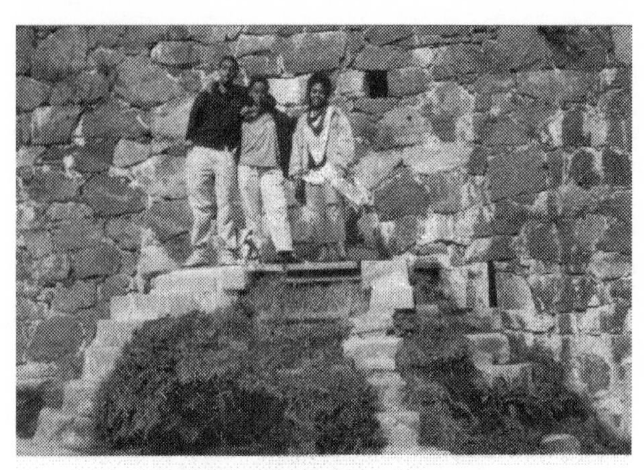

Abi with his sisters

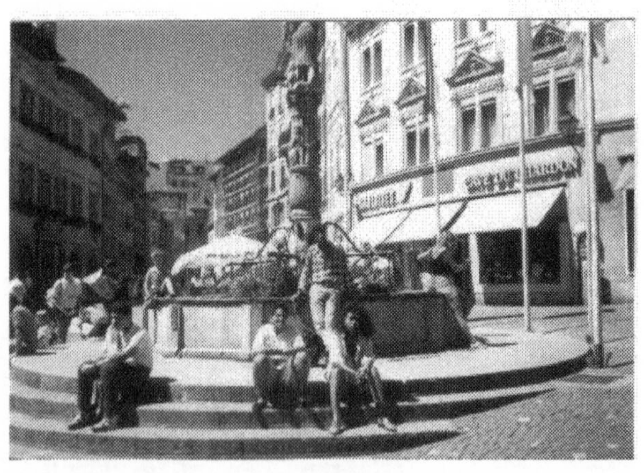

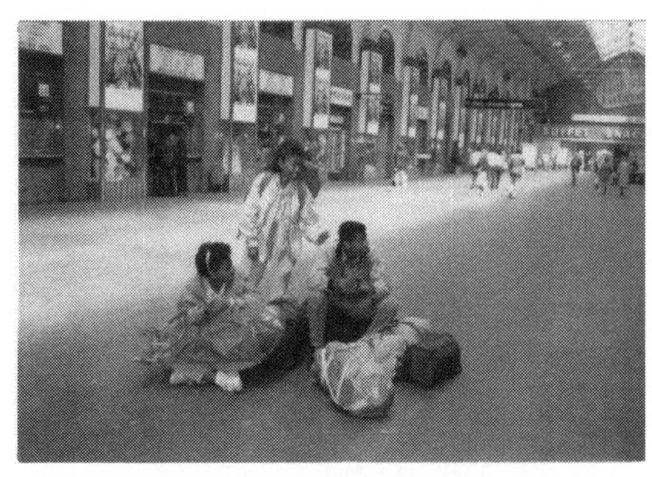

Abi with his sisters

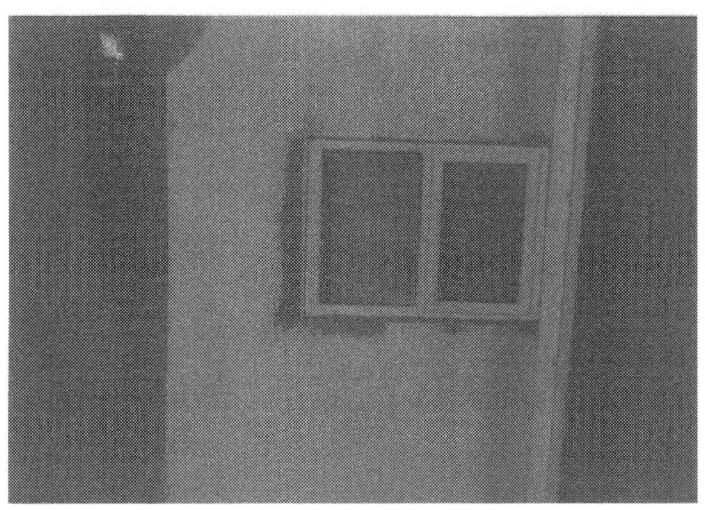

The bed sit from where he lived in solitude

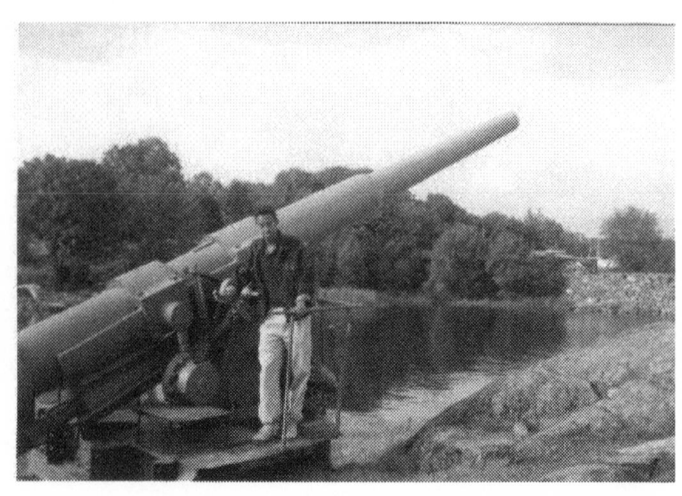

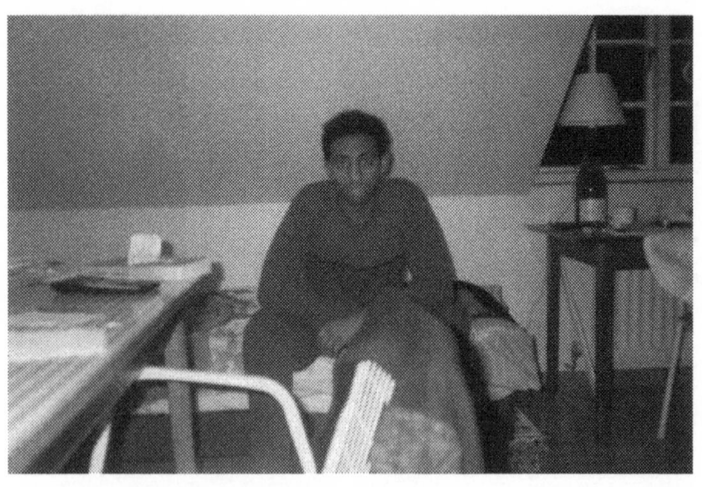

Abi - January 1988

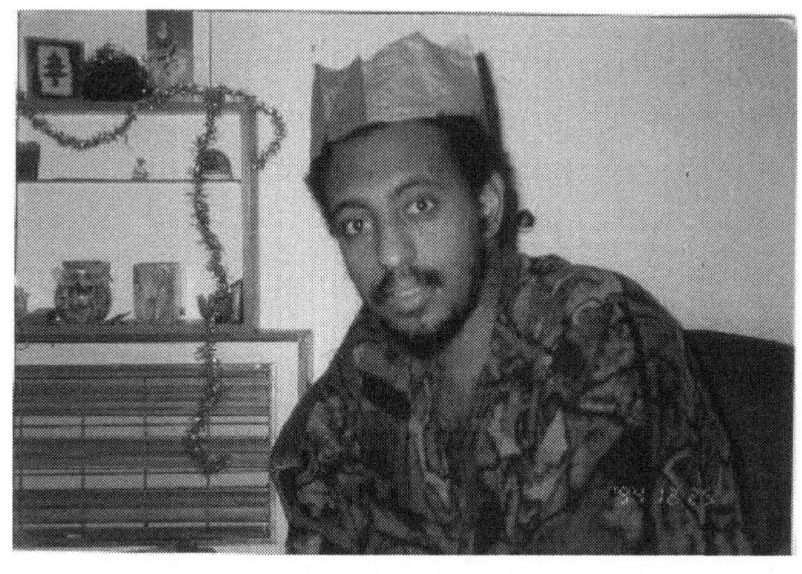

Abi - Christmas 1994 - His favorite Hymn
"Tell Out My Soul, the glory of the Lord"

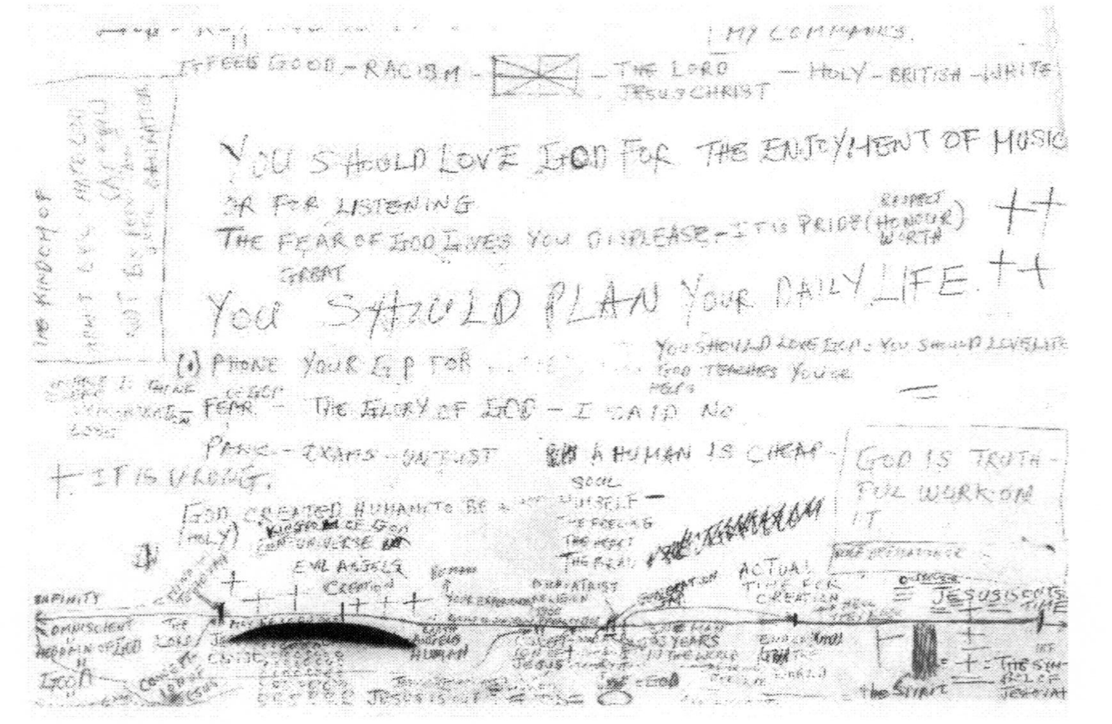

MY COMMANDS.
IT FEELS GOOD - RACISM - - THE LORD JESUS CHRIST - HOLY - BRITISH - WHITE
YOU SHOULD LOVE GOD FOR THE ENJOYMENT OF MUSIC
OR FOR LISTENING
THE FEAR OF GOD GIVES YOU DISPLEASE - IT IS PRIDE (RESPECT HONOUR WORTH)
YOU SHOULD PLAN YOUR DAILY LIFE.
(1) PHONE YOUR G.P FOR
FEAR - THE GLORY OF GOD - I SAID NO
PANIC - EXAMS - UNJUST
A HUMAN IS CHEAP
IT IS WRONG.
GOD CREATED HUMAN TO BE
GOD IS TRUTH-FUL WORK ON IT
EVIL ANGELS
ACTUAL TIME FOR CREATION
INFINITY
OMNISCIENT
THE START

DR. D. ATKINSON
DR. N. S. McCRAITH
DR. P. J. BERENDS-SHERIFF
DR. E. I. J. BUCKLEY
Consultation by appointment

St. Mary's Health Centre
Cop Lane
Penwortham
Preston
PR1 0SR
Tel: (0772) 744404

24 NOV 1993

Re Tefera Haile-Giorgis
53 Adelphi Place
Preston.

I can confirm that I first saw Tefera in Sept 1991 and that he was suffering from a severe anxiety and depression state.
It was arranged for Tefera to see a Psychiatrist urgently
His symptoms persist to date.

P. J. Berends-Sheriff

FOR SOCIAL SECURITY AND STATUTORY SICK PAY PURPOSES ONLY

Special Statement by the Doctor

In confidence to Mr/Mrs/Miss/Ms Teferra Haile-Giorgis

(A) I examined you on the following dates ....

....

....

and advised you that you should refrain from work

(B) I have not examined you but, on the basis of a recent written report from –

Doctor Devaraj ..... (Name if known)

of Royal Preston Hosp. S. G. Lane .... (Address)

I have advised you that you should refrain

from 27.12.94 to 19.1.95 from work for/until ....

Diagnosis of your disorder causing absence from work Depression.

Doctor's remarks DUPLICATE.

Doctor's signature [signature]

Date of signing 10.4.95

The special circumstances in which this form may be used are described in the handbook "Medical Evidence for Social Security and Statutory Sick Pay Purposes".

LANCASHIRE Family Practitione Committee
Dr. R. T. DAS 335655
34 Ashton Street, Preston PR2 2PP
Tel. 726508

Form Med 5 3/83

PATIENT TO COMPLETE PARTICULARS ON REVERSE

twelve hours after his father in Ethiopia. We do not know to this date whether Abi had found out about his father before he made his decision to end his life. A week after his father's burial Abi's body was flown from London to Addis Abeba and he was buried on the 28th of September 1996.

Unfortunately, we have not been able to find out precisely, from the hospital, how Abi managed to leave the hospital and find his way to the center of Preston. The coroner's report ruled that no one would be held accountable for Abi's death. In the cloud of uncertainty behind Abi's death, God has given us the strength to accept and heal from his tragic death. The journey to healing has been long but we believe that only God can provide such peace despite of lack in explanations.

During the time of our questioning we did not know of any groups in the United Kingdom which give support to families who, as a result of political and social difficulties, have suffered mental health problems.

This gap in care concerns us as a family and we are now in the process of finding a way of honoring Abi's own concern for those who suffer mentally due to circumstances of political conflict, imprisonment and displacement. We felt that a way in which we could remember Abi would be to set up a Trust which would enable us, in a small way, to stand by those who are suffering from mental health problems. A step towards the setting up of the Trust would be to commission a research of what already exists, in the United Kingdom,

for those who are mentally ill as a result of the political victimization, imprisonment and inevitable displacement.

We are hoping that the opportunity given to us by the Ethiopian Orthodox Church tradition of remembering the seventh year of death, will enable us to share with all those who are concerned about Abi's death, his life and the lives of many who have, and continue to suffer from mental illness as a result of circumstances for which they are not responsible. God's faithfulness to us as a family and His constant provision of healing for our loss inspires us to say:

"....and this, mortal shall have put on
immortality, shall be brought to pass the
saying that is written,
Death is
swallowed up in victory
"Where, O death, is your victory?
"Where, O death, is your sting? (1
Corinthians 15:54 and 55)
"But thanks be to God! He gives us the victory through our Lord Jesus Christ".
(1 Corinthians 15:57)

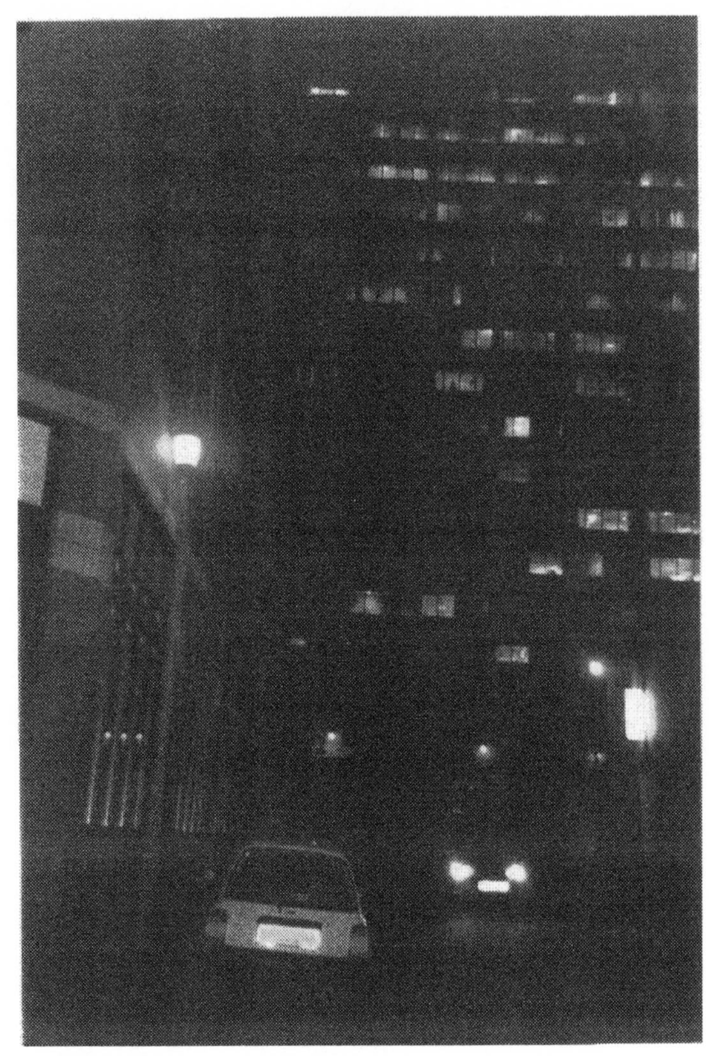

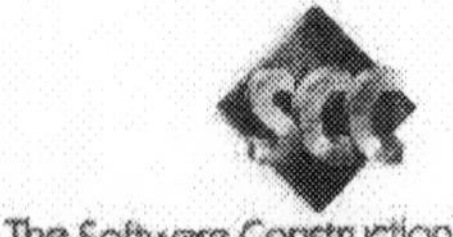

Library: **BRS TEXT LIBRARY** Record ID: **117258**

Headline
Byline
Body Text AN Ethiopian man died after plunging almost 100 feet from the **Guild Centre** in Preston.
Teferra Georgis, 26, was found dead on the pavement on Church Row outside
the **Guild** Centre offices on Friday afternoon at 3.50pm.
Mr Georgis was a psychiatric patient at the Royal Preston Hospital and staff reported having last seen him in the Avondale Unit just 10 minutes before he was found dead.
Content Date 23/9/96
Publication Lancashire Evening Post
Edition
Page
Category Gen
Keywords
Caption

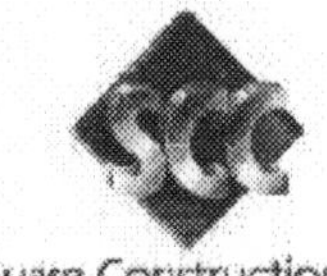

Library: **BRS TEXT LIBRARY**

Record ID: **117333**

Headline

Byline

Body Text AN INQUEST opened today into the death of an Ethiopian man who plunged
from the 15th floor of the **Guild Centre** offices in Preston.
The hearing was told Teferra Haile-Giorgis, 26, of Adelphi Street, was a psychiatric patient at Royal Preston Hospital and had been seen at the Avondale Unit minutes before he died.
He suffered from depression and obsessive behaviour and was found dead on
the pavement on Church Row at around 3.50pm on Friday.
County coroner Howard McCann adjourned the hearing for further medical
reports.

Content Date 25/9/96

Publication Lancashire Evening Post

Edition

Page

Category Gen

Keywords

Caption

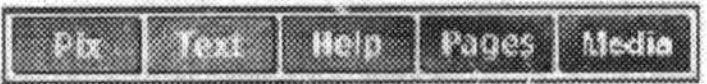

Pix | Text | Help | Pages | Media

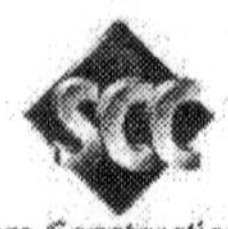

The Software Construction Company

Library: **BRS TEXT LIBRARY** Record ID: 118748

Headline
Byline
Body Text A MAN suffering mental health problems died after plunging 15-storeys from a Preston office block on the day his father died, an inquest heard.
County Coroner Howard McCann recorded an open verdict on Teferra Haile
Giorgis after hearing no suicide note was left and no-one saw how he fell from the top of the town centre building.
Mr **Giorgis** had a flat in Adelphi Street in Preston, but at the time of his death was resident at the Sycamore Ward of the Royal Preston Hospital's Avondale Unit.
After his death on Friday September 20 it was discovered that Mr Giorgis'
father had died that morning, but it was not known whether the news had been broken to him.
In his personal effects around 40 cash was discovered along with a note saying "Please give to the poor", but Mr McCann ruled this could not be counted as a suicide note.
Mr **Giorgis** was undergoing treatment because of the religious delusions he
suffered, the hearing heard.
On the day of his death he had been seen using a payphone on Sycamore ward just before he disappeared at about 3pm.
He was next seen an hour later by security staff at the Guild Centre offices near the bus station in Preston town centre.
Building manager Adrian Molloy spotted Mr **Giorgis** on the first floor, taking a lift to the uppermost 15th storey.
Dr Patrick Lynch, consultant pathologist at Royal Preston Hospital, said Mr **Giorgis** died from multiple injuries.
Mr McCann said: "We cannot interpret the note as suicide and no-one saw
him climb or fall out of the window, so I can only record an open verdict."
Content Date 13/11/96
Publication Lancashire Evening Post
Edition
Page
Category Gen
Keywords
Caption

D. Cert.
S.R./R.B.D.

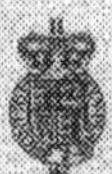

CAUTION—It is an offence to falsify a certificate or to make or knowingly use a false certificate or a copy of a false certificate intending it to be accepted as genuine to the prejudice of any person or to possess a certificate knowing it to be false without lawful authority.

CERTIFIED COPY OF AN ENTRY
Pursuant to the Births and Deaths Registration Act 1953

DEATH		Entry No. 231
Registration district Preston and South Ribble		Administrative area County of Lancashire
Sub-district Preston and South Ribble		
1. Date and place of death Twentieth September 1996 Church Row. Preston		
2. Name and surname Teferra HAILE-GIORGIS	3. Sex Male	4. Maiden surname of woman who has married —
5. Date and place of birth 28 July 1970 Ethiopia		
6. Occupation and usual address — Flat 5. 12-14 Adelphi Street Preston Lancs		
7.(a) Name and surname of informant Certificate received from M. H. McCann	(b) Qualification Coroner for Preston and South West Lancashire. Inquest held 12 November 1996	
(c) Usual address —		
8. Cause of death 1a Multiple Injuries Verdict:— Open Verdict		
9. I certify that the particulars given by me above are true to the best of my knowledge and belief —		Signature of informant
10. Date of registration Twelfth November 1996	11. Signature of registrar [illegible] Registrar	

Pat Nightingale,
21, Renshaw Drive
Walton-le-Dale
Preston
PR5 4RA.

21.9.96

To all Teferra's family

May I offer my deepest sympathy in your great loss, you have lost a son/~~father~~ brother/husband/father.

I have lost a friend. it was a pleasure knowing Teferra. We had a bumpy ride over the years but it was fun.

You brought up a lovely son who cared a lot about the human race, he was very well liked and I will miss him greatly even though many times we did not agree with each other. Perhaps now he has got his wish and is with his "Maker" and his father. Now he is at peace and nothing can harm him.

I will never ever know why he chose the route he did but that was his choice.

May he rest in peace.

I will pray for him.

God bless you all
always in my
thoughts.

Pat
x x x

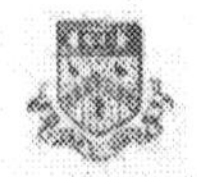

From the Headmaster
Dean Close School, Cheltenham, Glos. GL51 6HE
Telephone 522640 (Study)
Telephone [illegible] (Home)

5/11/96

My Dear Jembet and Workneh,

I was so sorry to hear of your devastating news from both Liz and Susan and I write to say how much you have been in Jill + my thoughts and prayers in recent weeks. I had trouble in getting the address – hence the delay.

I pray that the Lord of the Resurrection will Himself give you His comfort as you lean on Him. How hard the Evil One fights as we go forward in Jesus' work & how good to know that he will not have dominion for all power is given to our Saviour who came to destroy his works. May you know these truths deep in your hearts & may they sustain you for the next steps in His Service.

Dean Close continues well & we have much blessing in all ways. If you can come & see us, it will be a joy.

Very much love – Grace & Peace

Christopher

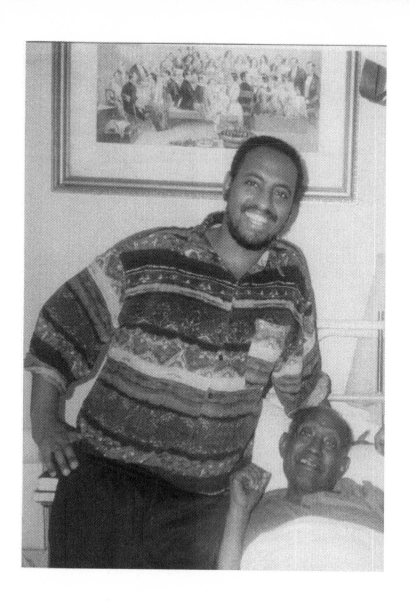

Flat 4
1 Portman Place
London E2 0LH

24th October 1996

O'Donnells Solicitor
68 Glovers Court
Preston PR1 3LS

Dear Mr O'Donnell

Thanks for your letter dated the 7th of October confirming your interest in representing my family at my brothers inquest. I can confirm that the corner has set a date for the hearing on Tuesday the 12th November at 9.45 am.

As per our discussion from our last meeting my family's aim form the inquest is to ascertain in detail with satisfactory reasoning the final days of my brothers life. In particular the last ten days before his death, we want to be satisfied that the care he has received form the Guild Trust for over three years has been maintained to the fullest until his death on the 20th of September without vindicating any individuals. In this process if the system is found to have any shortcomings in treating a unique cases like my brother's we wish it to be highlighted to the corner for a strong recommendation to the appropriate body so that to prevent something like this from happening ever again at the Avondale Unit or any other unit in the country.

From your letter you have quoted a figure in the region of £500 plus VAT for your services. Would it be possible for you to give me a break down of your charge with the view of the objectives we are trying to achieve form this inquest as soon as you are able to do so. This mighty enables us to budget the cost for the inquest in a better way especially if the figure above is only a preliminary estimate.

Lastly I will like to thank you for your continued interest in my brother's case and I know he would have appreciated your involvement in this proceedings. And we can hope this inquest will be beneficial for those who are involved in caring for the mentally ill in the future.

Hoping to hear form you very soon.

Yours sincerely

Workneh Hailegiorgis

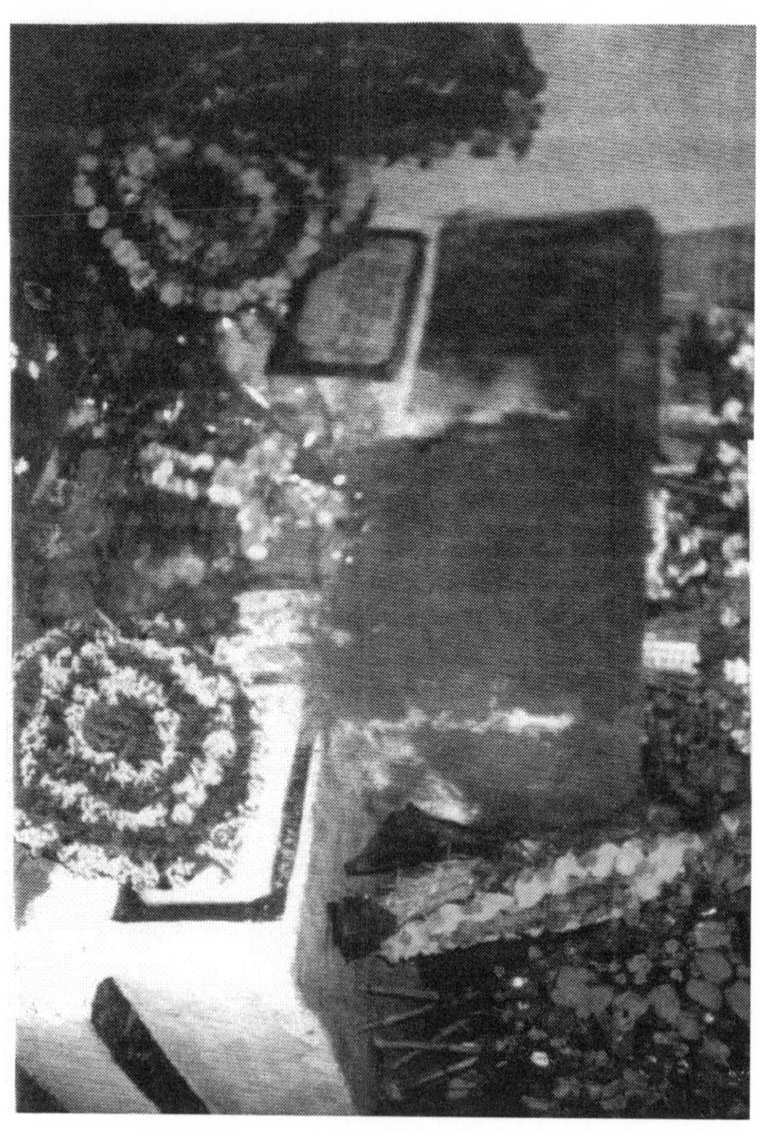

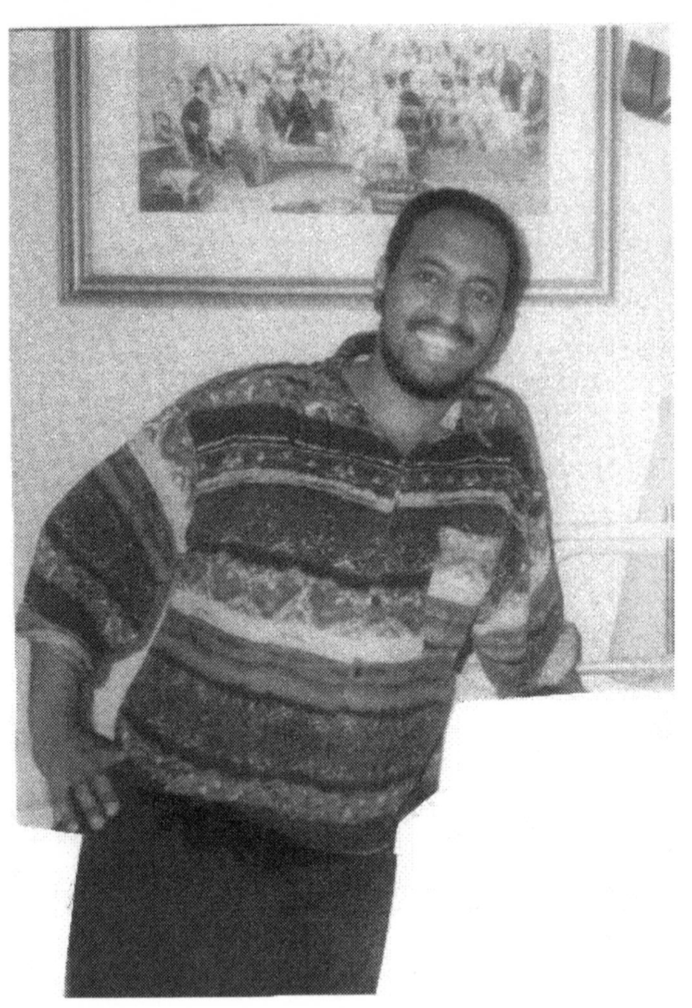

Lightning Source UK Ltd.
Milton Keynes UK
UKHW010823151222
413970UK00001B/330